Oral Embryology and Microscopic Anatomy

Figure 1. A photomicrograph of a ground section cut faciolingually through a human maxillary first premolar tooth. The enamel has a deep fissure in the central developmental groove. At the entrance to the fissure, on the triangular ridge of the buccal cusp, there is a barely visible dark area which is probably the beginning of a caries lesion. There is no evidence of caries at the bottom of the fissure.

In the enamel on the buccal and on the lingual surfaces of the crown there may be faintly seen near the dentinoenamel junction the narrow light and dark areas which are the bands of Hunter-Schreger.

Notice the curvature of the dentinal tubules in the crown of the tooth. Notice the configuration of the pulp chamber: the pulp horn in the buccal cusp extends much farther occlusally than the pulp horn in the lingual cusp. The pulp cavity here is empty because the pulp tissue was destroyed in the preparation of the section. Notice the relatively narrow root canals. It is difficult to distinguish the thickness of the cementum on this section at this magnification. (As seen under very low power of the microscope.)

Figure 1

Oral Embryology and Microscopic Anatomy

A Textbook for Students in Dental Hygiene

BY DOROTHY PERMAR, B.S., M.S.

*Professor of Dentistry (Oral Histology and Dental Anatomy),
College of Dentistry, The Ohio State University, Columbus, Ohio*

Fifth Edition

131 ILLUSTRATIONS

Lea & Febiger   Philadelphia

First Edition, 1955

Second Edition, 1959

Third Edition, 1963

Fourth Edition, 1967

  Reprinted, August, 1969

Fifth Edition, 1972

  Reprinted, June, 1973

ISBN: 0–8121–0376–9

Library of Congress Catalog Card Number: 70–170737

Printed in The United States of America

Published in Great Britain by Henry Kimpton Publishers, London

Preface

It is my hope that students of Dental Hygiene will find this textbook simple enough to be understandable and comprehensive enough to be useful.

The subject matter includes the embryonic development of the face and oral cavity; tooth enamel, dentin, cementum, and pulp; periodontal ligament and supporting bone; oral mucosa and salivary glands; development of teeth and their eruption, and in the case of primary teeth, their shedding. To this edition has been added a discussion and illustrations of dental caries and of developmental tooth anomalies. And, in response to suggestion, a chapter on the temporomandibular joint.

Mention is made of recent research in some aspects of oral histology; it is important that we should all be aware that what we learn as fact is not necessarily conclusive for all time. But it has seemed better to avoid lengthy discussion. The beginning student has so much to learn, in so many fields, that to confront him with accounts of conflicting results of numerous investigations which he has no background to analyze would not serve to broaden his education. It is rather for the advanced student to follow man's slow and often stumbling steps toward learning.

It is assumed that the student who uses this book has had a course in biology, and has some knowledge of both mammalian anatomy and human tooth morphology. Although it would be helpful, comprehensive instruction in histology or embryology is not necessary to this study.

This book is intended to be used in conjunction with lectures or discussion periods.

To the many students from whom I learn so much, I say "Thank you" for being so persevering. And particularly, "Thank you" to Dr. Bernard S. Snyder for the valuable supply, over many years, of extracted teeth which, throughout teaching of oral histology and dental anatomy, and for the illustrations in this book, have been the specimens for study of tooth morphology and microscopic anatomy. I greatly appreciate the generosity of Dr. Dennis Foreman for permitting me to use the electron micrograph of enamel rods (Fig. 20) and for his interpretation of the picture. Also I thank Dr. Rudy Melfi for Figures 2 and 131; Dr. Duncan McConnell for assistance in photography; Mr. Ralph Ulbrich for photography of the skull and many teeth; Miss Maureen Shalf for drawing Figure 82 and for other helpful assistance; Miss Marcelle Lasko for drawing Figure 129; and Mrs. Marice Kersey Musgrove for her friendly persuasion in the undertaking of this book.

DOROTHY PERMAR

Columbus, Ohio

Contents

11. TOOTH DEVELOPMENT

12. TOOTH ERUPTION AND THE SHEDDING OF THE PRIMARY TEETH

13. TEMPOROMANDIBULAR JOINT

Embryonic Development of the Face and Oral Cavity

THE HUMAN BODY

THE BEGINNING OF A HUMAN BODY

Beginning of life for an individual human being is the moment the sperm unites with the ovum and forms a fertilized egg. This egg divides into two cells, each of these into two more, and the resulting cells divide again and again. At first there is only a mass of but slightly differentiated cells; then begins a shaping—a shaping that eventually results in the formation of a tiny tubular embryo that foreshadows the plan of the adult human body.

An adult body is essentially a thick-walled tube. Or perhaps it can be better described as two tubes, a large outer one (outside body wall) and a small inner one (digestive tract), between which is a space (body cavity) that contains the internal organs: heart, lungs, liver. The mouth is the *cephalic* (head) opening of the inner tube, and the anus is the *caudal* (tail) opening.

Similarly in the tiny embryo, the tube which is the outside body wall encases a smaller tube, the *primitive digestive tract*, or *primitive gut*, which at this time is closed at both ends because the mouth and anus have not yet formed. In early stages of development, before the internal organs are formed, cells located between the outer body wall and the primitive digestive tract make the wall of the tubular embryo relatively thick.

In fact, the embryo wall is made up of three layers: *ectoderm* (ecto = outside; derm = skin); *mesoderm* (meso = middle); and *endoderm* (endo = inside). Collectively, these layers are called *primary embryonic layers*, or *primary germ layers*, and each is destined to form certain organs, or parts of organs, of the adult body. For example, ectoderm will give rise not only to the epithelium covering the outside of the body, but to the epithelium lining the oral cavity, nasal cavity, and sinuses, and to the enamel of the teeth, and to the nervous system. For the most part, from mesoderm will be derived the skeletal system, muscles, blood and lymph cells and vessels, kidneys, and some other internal organs, and also the dentin, cementum, and pulp of the teeth. And from endoderm will come the epithelial lining of the pharynx, stomach, and intestines, and of the lungs, bladder, vagina, and urethra.

From these three primary embryonic layers the manner of formation of the facial and oral structures will become clear as we study the embryonic development of the face and oral cavity, and later the development of the teeth.

Figure 2. *A and B.* A human embryo 25 mm. long—eight to nine weeks old. The head is large, making up nearly half of the body length. Compared to the size of the brain, the face appears small. The eyes are widespread; the ears are close to the neck. The nose is nearly flat. Notice the small size of the mandible. Inside of the mouth of an embryo of this age the lateral palatine processes are in a vertical position and the tongue is tall and narrow and nearly touches the lower border of the nasal septum (Fig. 7A). (Courtesy Dr. Rudy Melfi.)

The Size of a Human Fetus

At the end of the third week after fertilization the embryo is about 3 millimeters long. In later stages of development the size usually is given in terms of crown-rump length. By the end of the second month the crown-rump length is about 23 millimeters and the embryo has acquired a form recognizable as a human being (Fig. 2). At three months the fetus* has a crown-rump length of about 56 millimeters, and at four months about 112 millimeters.

THE DEVELOPMENT OF THE FACE

The Establishment of the Primitive Mouth

Throughout embryonic development the cephalic end of the embryo evolves in advance of the caudal end. The face starts to develop during the third week *in utero* with the beginning of the formation of the mouth, and by the end of the third week the *stomodeum*† (*primitive mouth*) has been established. It forms in this manner:

On the ventral side of the cephalic end of the embryo there occurs an invagination, an apparent pushing in, of the ectoderm. This depression is the *stomodeum* (Fig. 3). At the deepest part of this invagination the ectoderm is in contact with the endoderm of the *foregut* (the cephalic part of the primi-

---

* The unborn child is called an *embryo* until the end of the third month, after which time it is called a *fetus*.

† Pronounced *stō mō dē′ um*.

PLATE I

DEVELOPMENT OF THE HUMAN FACE

A and **B**. Human embryo, third week: Maxillary processes have developed from the first branchial arch. Stomodeum has formed. Frontal process (which here is blue) is undivided. Second and third branchial arches are visible. Depression on top of head is the neuropore. **C**. Fourth week: Nasal pits have divided the frontal process into the median nasal process (blue) and the right and left lateral nasal processes (pink).

stomodeum is lost. The posterior lobe of the hypophysis has a different origin; it is derived from the brain.

Now on the outside of the head, above and below the stomodeum opening, structures appear which will give rise to the face and to the various parts of the oral and nasal cavities.

Above the stomodeum the recently developed forebrain causes a large bulge (Figs. 3 and 4). The ectoderm and mesoderm that make up the surface of this bulge develop into an embryonic structure called the *frontal process* which will give rise to the upper part of the face, the nasal septum, and the anterior part of the roof of the mouth. The frontal process is shown in blue in Figure A of Plate I.

Below the stomodeum, in the region of the future neck, are formed five paired structures called *branchial arches*. These are ordinarily designated as branchial arches I, II, III, IV, and V (Fig. 4). In the development of the face and oral cavity only the first three arches play a part: branchial arch I develops into the mandible and a large part of the maxilla, and branchial arches II and III join the first branchial arch in the development of the tongue. Branchial arch I is shown in yellow in Figure A of Plate I.

And so by the end of the fourth week *in utero* the picture is this: The stomodeum has been established and the buccopharyngeal membrane has ruptured. Above the stomodeum is the frontal process, and immediately below it is the first branchial arch (Fig. 3). Excepting the base of the tongue, which is

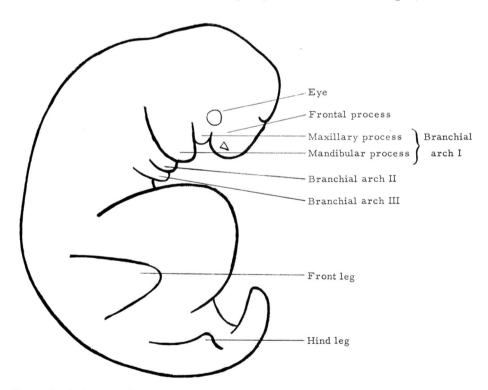

Figure 4. A drawing of a lateral view of a pig embryo. This is similar to human development at about six weeks *in utero*. Branchial arches IV and V are not visible here.

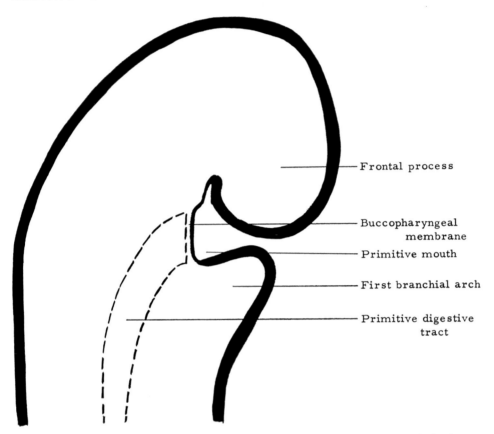

Frontal process

Buccopharyngeal
membrane

Primitive mouth

First branchial arch

Primitive digestive
tract

Figure 3. A diagrammatic illustration of a median sagittal section through the head of a human embryo at the end of the third week *in utero*. About 3 mm.

tive digestive tract). There is no intervening mesoderm. This combined ectoderm and endoderm is the *buccopharyngeal membrane*. (Examine Figure 3 carefully.) It is located approximately in the region where the palatine tonsils will later appear, and it separates the primitive mouth from the foregut. The location of the buccopharyngeal membrane indicates that the stomodeum is lined with ectoderm, and that the primitive digestive tract caudal to the stomodeum is lined with endoderm (Fig. 3).

During the fourth week *in utero* the buccopharyngeal membrane ruptures, and there is thus established communication between the stomodeum and the primitive digestive tract.

Shortly before the rupture of this membrane, at about the end of the third week *in utero*, begins the formation of a structure not usually thought of as being associated with the oral cavity. On the roof of the primitive mouth just in front of the buccopharyngeal membrane a small area of the stomodeal ectoderm evaginates (Fig. 3). The pit, known as *Rathke's pouch*, thus formed in the stomodeum roof deepens toward the brain, and these ectoderm cells from the stomodeum proliferate and develop into the *anterior lobe of the hypophysis*. The connection between the gland (anterior lobe of the hypophysis) and the

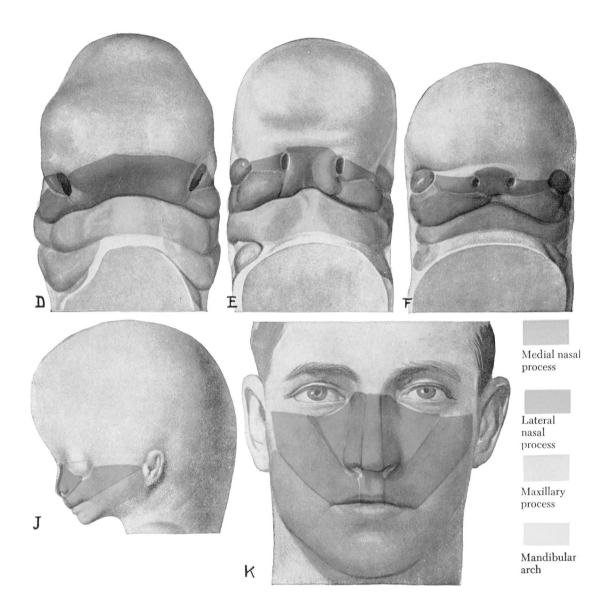

Medial nasal
process

Lateral
nasal
process

Maxillary
process

Mandibular
arch

D. Fifth week: Globular processes have appeared and are fused with the maxillary processes.
E. Sixth week: Due to differential growth, median nasal process is now relatively narrow. Eyes
are on lateral border of face. F. Seventh week: Median nasal process is relatively narrow.
Eyes are now anterior in position. G and H. Eighth week: Lidless eyes are on anterior of
face. The mandible is small. Nose protrudes slightly. Ears are low on side of head. I and J.
Twelfth week: Eyelids closed. Ears appear higher. Mandible further developed. K. Adult
face: Derivatives of median nasal process are blue; of lateral nasal processes are pink; of
maxillary processes are green; of mandibular processes are yellow.

(Sicher: *Orban's Oral Histology and Embryology*, courtesy of the C. V. Mosby Co.)

formed from branchial arches II and III, all of the face and all the structures of the oral and nasal cavities will now develop from these two *primary embryonic structures*—the *frontal process* and the *first branchial arch.*

EARLY DEVELOPMENT OF THE FACE

The development of the face centers about the mouth. After the establishment of the stomodeum, the frontal process, and the branchial arches, the next thing that happens is the budding of a rounded process on either end of the first branchial arch. These buds grow upward and medially (toward the center) at the right and left sides of the primitive mouth. They are the *maxillary processes* (Plate I, Figures A and B, green). After their appearance the remaining portion of the first branchial arch is called the *mandibular arch.* (Examine carefully Plate I, Figures A and B, yellow and green, and also Figures 4 and 5.) Eventually the maxillary processes will give rise to the upper part of the cheeks, the sides of the upper lip, and most of the palate. (Examine Plate I and follow the development of the maxillary processes, green, from Figures A and B to Figure K.) The mandibular arch will form the lower part of the cheeks, the mandible, and part of the tongue. (Examine Plate I and follow the development of the mandibular arch, yellow, from Figures A and B to Figure K.)

After the maxillary processes have formed, growth of the lower part of the face is retarded and the upper part of the face starts a rapid development. On the lower border of the frontal process appears a pair of depressions, the right and left *olfactory pits*, which are the future openings into the nose (Fig. 5 and Plate I, Figure C). The olfactory pits divide the lower part of the frontal process into three parts—a center portion called the *median nasal process*

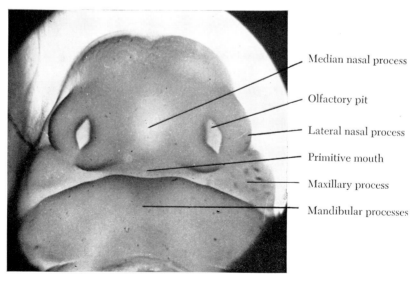

Median nasal process

Olfactory pit

Lateral nasal process

Primitive mouth

Maxillary process

Mandibular processes

Figure 5. A photograph of the face of a pig embryo of about 12 mm. At this stage of development the pig face and the human face are very much alike. (The *mandibular processes* are called the *mandibular arch.*)

(Plate I, Figure C, blue) and two lateral portions called the *right* and *left lateral nasal processes* (Plate I, Figure C, pink). The lateral nasal processes become the sides of the nose (Plate I, Figure K, pink), and the median nasal process forms the center and tip of the nose (Plate I, Figure K, blue). Later, an ingrowth from the median nasal process (the center of the nose) into the stomodeum forms the nasal septum (the division between the right and left nasal chambers).

At its lower border, the median nasal process now grows in length and produces a pair of bulges called the *globular process*. The globular process is not separated into two parts, but remains as a single median structure which grows downward so that it extends below the olfactory pits and lies between the right and left maxillary processes (Plate I, Figure E). It forms the center of the upper lip (the *philtrum*) (Plate I, Figures I and K, and also Figure 6), and during the formation of the interior of the mouth it gives rise to the anterior part of the palate, the premaxilla (Fig. 8).

LATER DEVELOPMENT OF THE FACE

In the course of facial development there is considerable *differential growth:* that is, some parts grow faster than other parts. These differences in the rate of growth result in marked progressive changes in the relative size and position of the various structures. Because of the rapid growth of surrounding areas, the slower growing median nasal process becomes relatively more narrow, and the nasal openings relatively closer together (Plate I, Figures C through I). The eyes, which appeared first on the sides of the head (Plate I, Figure E), due to differential growth come to be located on the front of the head (Plate I, Figure I), while the ears change in position from the neck region (Plate I, Figure H) to the sides of the head (Plate I, Figure K). For a time the relatively slow growth of the mandibular arch results in a lag in the development of the lower part of the face (Plate I, Figures G and H). The mandible of a two-month-old embryo (Fig. 2) is very small in proportion to the upper part of the face.

Along with the development of the various embryonic structures there occur fusions of certain of the processes. The only openings that remain in the fully formed face are the openings of the mouth and of the two nostrils, all other divisions between embryonic parts having been closed by fusions of one form or another.

Two lines of fusion occur in the upper lip. The right and left maxillary processes, which bud from the superolateral borders of the first branchial arch (Plate I, Figures A and B), grow forward and fuse with the right and left sides of the globular process. Thus the globular process forms the center of the upper lip, and the maxillary processes form the sides of the upper lip (Plate I, Figures D through K, and also Figure 6). The fusions in the upper lip are completed by the end of the second month *in utero*.

A partial or complete failure of fusion of a maxillary process with the globular process results in a condition known as *cleft lip* (Fig. 6). Cleft lip may be either unilateral or bilateral: that is, it may involve a failure of fusion of the globular process either with the right or with the left maxillary process, or

Figure 6. Diagram of an adult human face showing the derivations of its parts from the frontal process and the first branchial arch. *A* and *B* indicate the locations where clefts sometimes occur in the upper lip and in the mandible. (The *mandibular processes* are called also the *mandibular arch*.)

with both the right and the left maxillary processes. If a cleft of the lip occurs, it will be apparent by the end of the second month *in utero*, since that is the time that the fusions of the lip are ordinarily completed.

Fusion also occurs at the corners of the mouth between the maxillary processes and the mandibular arch. This decreases the breadth of the oral opening (Fig. 6). In the adult a line of yellowish spots frequently seen extending laterally along the inside of the cheek from either corner of the mouth is said to be evidence of these embryonic fusions. These small yellowish elevations, called *Fordyce's spots* (Chapter 9), are sebaceous glands. Sebaceous glands are expected, of course, only on the outside of the body, but are thought to have become entrapped here in the cheek at the time of fusion of the right and left maxillary processes with the right and left ends of the mandibular arch and to persist in the adult oral mucosa.

A failure of fusion at the corners of the mouth of the maxillary processes and the mandibular arch leaves a cleft which results in an exceptionally large mouth opening. This anomaly (deviation from the usual) is known as *macrostomia*.

Very early in the life of the embryo there is a filling in of the deep depression which originally separates the right and left sides of the mandibular arch at the midline (Plate I, Figure E). In the adult mandible evidence of the early existence of this depression may persist as a deep dimple in the chin. A failure of proper filling of this depression in the development of the embryo may result in a *median cleft* of the mandible (Fig. 6). This kind of cleft is rare.

Also rare is a cleft extending from the upper lip to the eye, called an *oblique facial cleft*. There are differing opinions about the manner of formation of a cleft in this location. Apparently it is not due to a failure of fusion of embryonic processes, but possibly to the failure of swellings of the maxillary process and the lateral nasal process to merge. The explanation of the mechanism of this developmental defect is at present not clear.

In the course of the fusion of completely separated embryonic processes, or of the filling in of grooves which partially separate embryonic structures, small areas of epithelial cells at the line of union may become surrounded, entrapped, and embedded. The presence of these *epithelial rests* accounts for the presence of cysts which are sometimes found in such locations as the upper lip on either side of the philtrum, in the cheek on a line with the corners of the mouth, in the midline of the chin, and, as we shall see later, in the roof of the mouth.

SUMMARY OF THE DEVELOPMENT OF THE FACE

The beginning of face development is seen in the human embryo during the third week *in utero* when an invagination of the ectoderm forms the *stomodeum*. Above the stomodeum is the *frontal process*, and below the stomodeum is the *first branchial arch*. Buddings on the superolateral border at either end of the first branchial arch form the *maxillary processes*, and the first branchial arch is thus divided into (1) two *maxillary processes* and (2) a *mandibular arch*. Invaginations on either side of the lower border of the frontal process, the *olfactory pits*, divide the frontal process into the *median nasal process* and *right and left lateral nasal processes*. The median nasal process grows downward and produces the *globular process*. The lateral nasal processes become the sides of the nose. The right and left maxillary processes grow medially from the corners of the primitive mouth and beneath the nose they fuse with the globular process to form the upper lip. At the corners of the primitive mouth fusion of the maxillary processes with the mandibular arch reduces the size of the broad oral opening. Early in development the midline depression in the mandibular arch disappears. *Differential growth* results in, among other things, a movement of the eyes from the sides of the head to the front of the head and of the ears from the neck to the sides of the head. By the end of the second month *in utero* most of these developments have taken place. The mandible is still relatively underdeveloped.

Clefts which sometimes occur in the face as a result of faulty development include cleft lip, cleft chin, oblique facial cleft, and clefts at the corners of the mouth.

THE DEVELOPMENT OF THE ORAL CAVITY AND NASAL CAVITY

THE DEVELOPMENT OF THE PALATE AND NASAL SEPTUM

The palate (the roof of the mouth) shows marked development near the end of the second month *in utero*. It arises from three sources: from the *right* and the *left maxillary processes* and from the *globular process*. It forms in this

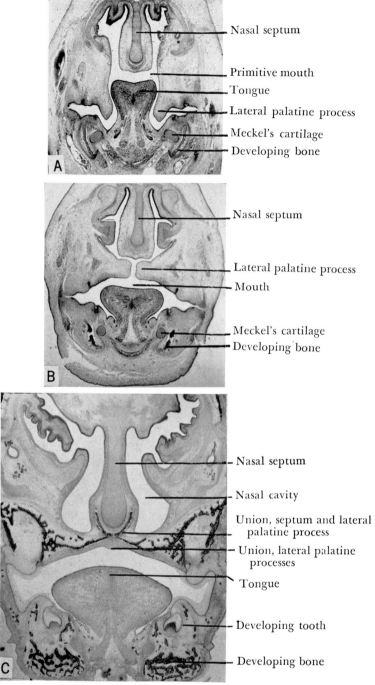

Nasal septum

Primitive mouth

Tongue

Lateral palatine process

Meckel's cartilage

Developing bone

A

Nasal septum

Lateral palatine process

Mouth

Meckel's cartilage

Developing bone

B

Nasal septum

Nasal cavity

Union, septum and lateral
palatine process

Union, lateral palatine
processes

Tongue

Developing tooth

Developing bone

C

Figure 7. Frontal sections through the head of 3 pigs showing progressive stages in development of the palate. This is similar to human palatal development. A. The vertical position of the lateral palatine processes and the position of the tongue which nearly touches the lower border of the nasal septum are similar to the condition in an eight-week-old human embryo (Fig. 2). B. The shortening and broadening of the tongue, the horizontal position of the palatine processes, and their lack of union at the midline are similar to the condition in a nine-week-old human embryo. C. In a human fetus of twelve weeks, as in this pig fetus, the palatine processes have fused with each other and with the lower border of the nasal septum. The oral cavity and the nasal cavity are now separated by the roof of the mouth.

9

way: Inside the stomodeum, near the end of the second month, appear three ingrowths. One is from the inner surface of the right maxillary process, one is from the inner surface of the left maxillary process, and one is from the inner surface of the globular process. (Examine Plate I, Figure H, and notice the extent of the maxillary processes, green; and in Figure G, the centrally located globular process, blue.) The ingrowths into the stomodeum from the inside of the maxillary processes are called the *right* and *left lateral palatine processes*. The ingrowth from the globular process becomes the *premaxilla* (Fig. 8). It originates first as the bar of tissue, called the *primary palate*, located inside the stomodeum between and a little beneath the right and left olfactory pits. This is about the place where the globular process arises from the median nasal process. Further ingrowth into the stomodeum from this area develops into the *premaxilla*. The eventual union of the two maxillary processes with each other and with the premaxilla (Fig. 8) will close the Y-shaped opening in the roof of the mouth.

In the course of union, or fusion, of these palatal structures the developing tongue becomes strangely involved. The tongue begins to develop at the end of the first month *in utero*. By the end of the second month, when the lateral palatine processes appear, the tongue is a comparatively large organ which extends upward in this primitive cavity until its upper surface nearly touches the lower border of the nasal septum (Fig. 7A). At first the newly developing right and left lateral palatine processes grow not horizontally, but rather they grow downward to the right and left of the elevated tongue (Fig. 7A).

The determinant of the subsequent lifting of these processes to a horizontal

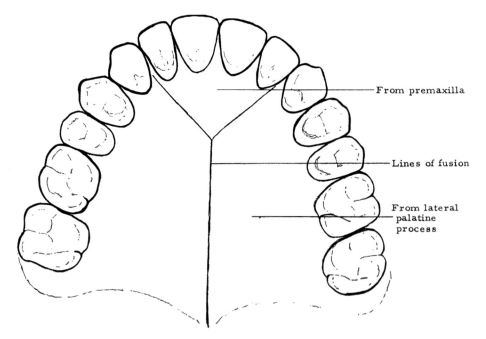

Figure 8. Drawing of the oral surface of a human maxilla.
The Y-shaped lines of embryonic fusion are indicated.

position (Fig. 7*B*) has been the subject of much careful study. A frequent explanation is that as a result of enlargement of the mandible and a change in the degree of flexion of the fetus head, the tongue drops to the floor of the stomodeum; and when the tongue is thus removed from the path of the growing lateral palatine processes, the processes are straightened to a horizontal position by a sort of hinge movement, the causative force being, perhaps, rapid cell division at their lateral borders.

Change in position from vertical to horizontal of the lateral palatine processes occurs rapidly. In the mouse embryo this elevation has been found to take only a few hours, and apparently it is correspondingly rapid in the human embryo. Studies of this action have been extremely interesting, but have not yet supplied a clear explanation of the mechanism of this palatal movement. *

Having attained a horizontal position early in the third month, the lateral palatine processes grow medially, toward each other (Fig. 7*B*), and the developing premaxilla grows posteriorly. The palatine processes meet at the midline and fuse with each other and with the lower border of the nasal septum (Fig. 7*C*); and at their anterior borders they meet and fuse with the posterior border of the premaxilla (Fig. 8). The structure thus formed is at once the roof of the oral cavity and the floor of the nasal cavity: the stomodeum has been divided into a lower chamber and an upper chamber.

The critical period for the movement and complete closure of the lateral palatine processes and the premaxilla lies between eight and twelve weeks *in utero*. The fusions of the roof of the mouth are normally completed by the end of twelve weeks *in utero*.

The palatal fusions, at the time they occur, are fusions of soft tissue, not of bone. Small areas of forming bone tissue are first seen in the developing palate during the eighth week *in utero*, when the lateral palatine processes are still in a vertical position. By the end of the third month, when the embryonic palatal structures are completely fused, there is considerable bone tissue in the area, but the bones of the right and left sides of the hard palate are not together at the midline. A separation of the *bones* of the right and left sides of the roof of the mouth still exists at the end of the fourth month *in utero*.

During the time the roof of the mouth is forming, the nasal cavity becomes divided into a right and a left chamber by the nasal septum. This septum develops chiefly as a growth into the stomodeum from the inside of the median nasal process. (Examine Plate I, Figure G, and notice how an ingrowth on the median nasal process, blue, directed posteriorly and downward, would form a central partition of the part of the stomodeum that is becoming the nasal chamber.) When the right and left lateral palatine processes fuse with each other in the midline of the palate, they fuse also with the inferior border of the nasal septum (Fig. 7*C*).

As is true in any location where fusions of embryonic processes occur, in the lines of palatal fusion groups of epithelial cells, called *epithelial rests*, may become entrapped. These misplaced rudiments of epithelium are the origin of cysts that sometimes are found in the palatal area.

---

* Interesting paper: Walker, B. E.: Palate Morphogenesis in the Rabbit. Arch. Oral Biol. *16*:275, 1971.

Just as a failure of proper fusion of one or both maxillary processes with the globular process results in a cleft of the upper lip, a failure of the lateral palatine processes to fuse with each other or with the premaxilla results in a *cleft of the palate*. If cleft palate occurs, it will be apparent by the end of the third month *in utero*, since this is the time that the palatal fusions are ordinarily completed.

Cleft palate may be slight or extensive. It may involve only the uvula,* in which case it does not affect oral function. It may involve the soft palate, or a small part of the hard palate, or both the soft and hard palate. Cleft palate sometimes involves the alveolar ridge on one or both sides of the midline—that is, cleft of the alveolar ridge may be either unilateral or bilateral (Fig. 8). Often such a cleft is located between the maxillary lateral incisor and the canine teeth. Sometimes the lateral incisor is missing. In any kind of severe intraoral cleft the maxillary teeth may be incomplete in number, and often they are greatly misplaced. Any severe cleft of the palate produces a crippling opening between the oral and nasal cavities. This opening is a serious handicap to the individual in both speaking and eating. Cleft palate may occur with or without the presence of cleft lip.

A review of the literature on cleft lip and cleft palate in human beings† has revealed substantial evidence in support of the following conclusons:

Nearly 6,000 new cases of cleft lip and cleft palate occur each year in the United States.

Cleft lip, with or without associated cleft palate, is more common in boys than in girls (65:35 ratio).

Cleft palate is more common in girls than in boys (60:40 ratio).

Considering all types of clefts, boys are more frequently affected than girls (58:42 ratio).

Clefts of the lip occur more frequently on the left side than on the right. Over 61 per cent of unilateral clefts of the lip occur on the left side. No reason for this is at present known.

A *possible* explanation for the greater frequency of palatal clefts in girls than in boys was deduced from the study of 46 human embryos.‡ There seems to be a time lag in females compared to males in the change in position of the palatal processes from vertical to horizontal, and this may render females susceptible for a longer period of time to conditions which could interfere with palatal closure.

Strong indication exists that genetic factors can determine the occurrence of cleft palate. It has been found that in 20 to 30 per cent of affected children there is some family history of clefts, but a definite hereditary pattern has not been determined. Also, clefts have been induced in unborn rats and mice by events that occur *during the time of normal palatal closure*, such as the administration at this precise time of cortisone or of excessive vitamin A (or of a number of other things) to the pregnant female. This information obtained from animal studies cannot, of course, be applied directly to human development.

* The pendulum of soft tissue hanging down toward the base of the tongue from the center of the posterior border of the soft palate. Examine someone's mouth and see this structure.
† Greene, J. C.: Pub. Health Rep., 78:589, 1963.
‡ Burdi, A. R. and R. G. Silvey: The Cleft Palate Jour. 6, No. 1, 1–7, 1969.

The Development of the Tongue

Anatomically the tongue has a *body* (the anterior part) and a *root* (the posterior part). The body extends from the tongue tip to the *terminal sulcus*, which is the V-shaped groove on the top surface just behind a V-shaped row of circumvallate papillae (Fig. 82). (Examine someone's tongue as far back as you can see and find this row of papillae.) The root of the tongue lies behind the terminal sulcus. The tongue has been aptly described as a sac of mucous membrane filled with voluntary muscle.

When the embryo is four weeks old the tongue begins to develop from the anterior wall of the primitive throat, and protrudes upward and anteriorly. Embryologically it develops from the region of the first three branchial arches. To picture its development, imagine yourself standing in the throat of a human embryo at the beginning of the second month and facing forward. Before your eyes near the center line on the inner surface of the mandibular arch are recently formed *lingual swellings* which will unite and become a single structure, the body of the tongue. Behind these, in the center line between the second and third branchial arches, involving the inner ends of these arches, is a swelling which will become the base of the tongue. These swellings from the three branchial arches unite into the single organ which by the end of the second month *in utero* will have acquired a recognizable form and will extend upward and forward toward the opening of the mouth.

In the fully formed tongue behind the circumvallate papillae at the tip of the V-shaped line (Fig. 82) is a small depression, the *foramen caecum*, which marks the point of embryonic origin of the *thyroid gland*. At about seventeen days *in utero*, in the midline between the first and second branchial arches, the gland originates as a small proliferation of epithelium. As it develops, it descends to its final position in the neck, remaining attached to the tongue during its migration by a narrow *thyroglossal duct*. The duct eventually disappears, but the place of origin of the thyroid gland is marked on the tongue by the presence of the foramen caecum.

A rare deformity is a bifurcation of the body of the tongue. When this anomaly occurs it is probably because the lingual swellings of the first branchial arch failed to merge. Other possible anomalies are too large a tongue (macroglossia), too small a tongue (microglossia), and absence of a tongue (aglossia).

Summary of the Development of the Oral and Nasal Cavities

The *premaxillary region* of the *palate* develops from the *globular process*, a downward growth of the *median nasal process* which is the center part of the original *frontal process*. The sides of the palate are formed by the *lateral palatine processes*. These arise from the *maxillary processes*, which are buds from the ends of the *first branchial arch*. These three structures, the premaxilla and the right and the left palatine processes, fuse in the roof of the mouth in a Y-shaped pattern (Fig. 8). From the part of the frontal process which forms the center of the nose (the *median nasal process*), the *nasal septum* grows back and downward, and its inferior border fuses with the center of the hard palate.

The *tongue* develops as growths from the mid-anterior region on the inner surface of the *first three branchial arches:* the body of the tongue from the first branchial arch; the base from the second and third.

Clefts which sometimes occur inside the mouth as a result of faulty development include partial or complete clefts of the palatal structures, and cleft of the tongue.

SUMMARY OF THE DEVELOPMENT OF THE FACE AND ORAL CAVITY

A summary of the derivations of the structures of the face and oral cavity is presented in the following outline:

I. From the *Frontal Process* are derived:

    1. Median nasal process, which gives rise to:
        a. Center and tip of nose
        b. Nasal septum
        c. Globular process, which gives rise to:
            (1) Philtrum of upper lip
            (2) Premaxilla

    2. Lateral nasal processes, which form:
        a. Sides of nose
        b. Infraorbital areas

II. From *Branchial Arch I* are derived:

    1. Mandibular arch, which gives rise to:
        a. Mandible
        b. Lower parts of face
        c. Anterior part of tongue

    2. Maxillary processes, which give rise to:
        a. Lateral palatine processes (*i.e.,* all of palate and maxillary alveolar arch excepting premaxilla)
        b. Upper part of cheeks
        c. Sides of upper lip

III. From *Branchial Arches II and III* are derived portions of the posterior part of the tongue.

All of the face and most of the structures of the oral cavity develop from two primary embryonic structures: the *frontal process* and the *first branchial arch.* The tongue alone adds to its origin the second and third branchial arches.

CHAPTER 2

Introduction to Histology

GENERAL HISTOLOGY

THE NATURE OF HISTOLOGY

Histology is the science of tissues (histo = tissue; logy = the science of). Of particular interest in Dentistry are the tissues of the oral cavity.

A *tissue* is sometimes defined as a group of more or less similar cells with intercellular substance and tissue fluid, combined in a characteristic manner and performing a particular function. Some examples of human tissues are muscle, bone, blood, epithelium of the skin and of the mucous membrane, connective tissue of the skin and of the mucous membrane, and the pulp of a tooth. The hard components of a tooth, enamel, dentin, and cementum, are also tissues, although enamel and dentin, and some cementum, have exceptional characteristics.

Tissues vary greatly in appearance and in structure. Some are hard (bone); some are soft (muscle). Some are sturdy and withstand wear and injury (surface layer of the skin); and some are delicate and serve as linings (lining of the respiratory tract). Some are secretory in function (salivary gland tissue); and some are nutritive in function (blood).

HOW TISSUES ARE STUDIED

Microscopic examination of tissues started in the early nineteenth century, and study has been extended and developed as improvements have been made in the construction of microscopes and in the techniques of tissue preparation. Usually tissues must be stained in some manner in order that their different components may be seen clearly with a microscope. Sometimes dyes are injected into the blood stream of a living animal, and the tissues which have taken up the stain from the blood are subsequently removed from the animal and cut into thin sections. Or tissues may be grown in artificial nutrient media in a glass tube, and their growth and development observed from hour to hour or from day to day. The most usual method of tissue preparation is probably that of removing a small piece of tissue from the body, embedding it in paraffin, sectioning it, and staining it.

Let us suppose, for example, that a dentist wants to examine the microscopic structure of the soft tissue surrounding the teeth. A small piece of this gingival tissue is carefully removed from the mouth with a sharp instrument and is immediately placed in a bottle containing 10 per cent formalin. In this solution it is sent to a microtechnique laboratory. When the specimen is received in the laboratory, it is dehydrated in absolute alcohol, allowed to stand in

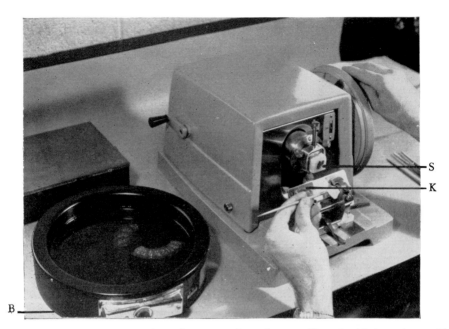

Figure 9. A rotary microtome is used to cut sections of a paraffin-embedded specimen. The dark-colored specimen (S), embedded in a block of white paraffin, is attached to the microtome. The knife (K) is in a horizontal position beneath the paraffin block. As the wheel is turned with the right hand, the block moves up and down behind the knife, advancing several microns with each cycle. Sections of the block come off in a ribbon, which is taken up with a brush held in the left hand. Short lengths of the ribbon of sections are floated on warm water in a constant temperature bath (B). Separated into strips of suitable length, the sections are lifted from the water by slipping a glass microscope slide under them.

xylene, and then placed in a dish of melted paraffin which is kept in a warming oven. In a few hours the paraffin will have completely permeated the tissue. The paraffin and tissue are then poured into a small paper container. Hardened in cool water, the paraffin becomes a firm block which contains the specimen in its center. The paraffin block is then cut into sections (slices) with an instrument called a microtome (Fig. 9). Each paraffin section is about 8 microns thick and has in its center, of course, a section of the embedded specimen which is the same in thickness. The paraffin sections are arranged on glass microscope slides, with egg albumin used as an adhesive. The slides are then passed through xylene which dissolves away the embedding paraffin, leaving the thin section of tissue attached to the slide. In order that the structure of the tissue may be studied, it is necessary now to pass the slides through appropriate tissue stains.

There are innumerable kinds of tissue stains. One of the common combinations of stains is hematoxylin and eosin. When the slides bearing the sections of tissue are immersed in the hematoxylin the nuclei of the cells will take up the stain and become deep blue. Subsequent immersion in the eosin stain will cause the cytoplasm of the epithelial cells to become a pinkish color and the intercellular substance of the connective tissue to become very pink. Stains other than hematoxylin and eosin are used to bring out different tissue structures. After they are stained the tissue sections are covered with a small, very thin cover glass. In this way the slides are permanently preserved.

Specimens which contain calcified tissue such as bone and teeth must be decalcified in a weak acid before they can be cut with the sharp knife of the microtome. The decalcification process is the removal (dissolving) of the mineral material from the organic material of a tissue. Five per cent nitric acid is often used for this purpose. As a result of this decalcification process, changes are inevitable in certain tissues. Tooth enamel, for instance, is usually entirely lost when a tooth is allowed to stand in acid. Tooth enamel is about 96 per cent mineral material and only 4 per cent organic material and water. When the mineral material is removed by the acid, the delicate organic portion of the enamel is mechanically washed away unless special techniques for its preservation are employed. Other kinds of calcified tissues retain their form when they are decalcified. Dentin, cementum, and bone, because they contain a much greater proportion of organic material, are not thus destroyed when the mineral material is removed in the process of decalcification. Completely decalcified dentin, cementum, or bone will retain its original shape, although it can be easily pierced with a needle.

The enamel of a tooth may be preserved for study if instead of using the decalcifying, embedding, and sectioning procedures the tooth is merely ground down to one thin section. This is done on a lathe with a revolving stone. With this technique it is not difficult to obtain a tooth section less than 20 microns thick. Specimens of teeth prepared in this way are referred to as *ground sections*. Ground sections are mounted on glass slides and covered with a cover glass in the same way that other types of sections are preserved

COMPONENTS OF A TISSUE

Tissues are made up of *cells, intercellular substance*, and *tissue fluid*.

A *cell* is a unit of living substance (protoplasm), usually having cytoplasm and a nucleus. It may exist as an individual, as in unicellular animals, or it may be part of a tissue of a large animal or plant and be dependent upon other cells for existence.

Cells show an almost infinite variation in size, shape, and structure. In animals the largest of cells is an ovum: a chicken egg, or even a human ovum (120 microns in diameter). In contrast to these cells, a human red blood cell is about 8 microns in diameter.

Circulating human red blood cells have lost their nuclei; white blood cells contain one or several nuclei. Muscle cells are distinctive because their cytoplasm has the power of strong contraction (Fig. 10 E and F). Fat cells contain large amounts of fat, which push the nuclei away from the center of the cells and against the cell walls. There are many kinds of cells which, along with varying kinds and amounts of intercellular substance and different amounts of tissue fluid, determine the nature of the various kinds of tissues.

Intercellular substance is a product of living cells and is distributed among the cells in all of the tissues of the body. It holds the cells together and provides a medium for the passing of nutrients and of waste materials from capillaries to cells and from cells to capillaries. The amount and kind of intercellular substance differ in different tissues. In some human tissues, such as bone, intercellular substance is the predominant element. In other human tissues, such as the epithelium which makes up the surface of the skin, intercellular substance is small in amount and the cellular elements predominate. Intercellular substance occurs in two forms: one form is *fibrous* in nature, and the other is *amorphous* in nature (a = without; morphous = form).

Tissue fluid is that part of the blood plasma which can diffuse through the walls of capillaries. In the tissue fluid nutrients are carried out through capillary walls to the surrounding intercellular substance and then to the cells; and waste products of the cells are returned in the same manner from the intercellular substance to the capillaries. Tissue fluid may be present in a tissue in relatively small proportions, as in the epithelium of the surface of the skin; or it may form a large proportion of the tissue, as in blood. The tissue fluid of epithelium, of bone, and of other tissues is, of course, derived from blood.

Classification of Tissues

In their gross and microscopic appearance, and in their function, tissues vary so widely that the beginning student may well feel that there is little or no relationship among them. This seeming confusion grows less, however, when it it discovered that for purposes of easier study and better understanding histologists have developed a classification for tissues. Tissues are alike in that they are made up of cells, intercellular substance, and tissue fluid. Tissues differ in the form and number of cells, in the type and amount of intercellular substance, and in the amount of tissue fluid. It is on the similarities and differences of tissues that the histologist has based his classification.

Human tissues have been assorted into *four primary groups: epithelial tissue, connective tissue, muscle tissue,* and *nerve tissue.* The tissues of each of these primary groups have certain major, fundamental characteristics in common. But there are also differences within the groups; and so each of the four primary groups has been subdivided. The subdivisions are based on structural differences which clearly distinguish one tissue from another.

A brief classification of human tissues is presented in Table 1.

Tissues are combined in characteristic ways to form organs, such as heart, lungs, liver, bones, skin, tongue; and organs are combined in characteristic ways to form organisms, such as the human body.

Let us consider the tongue as an organ. The tongue is made up of a combination of epithelial tissue, connective tissue, muscle tissue, and nerve tissue all of which are interdependent in the functioning of the organ (Fig. 11). Epithelial tissue comprises the surface of the tongue and serves as a protective covering. Beneath the epithelium is connective tissue which supplies both support and nourishment; and beneath this connective tissue layer are strong muscles which produce movement of the organ. Nerves of the tongue supply both motor and sensory functions.

Another organ of the human body is the skin. Skin is made up of a combination of epithelial tissue, connective tissue, and nerves. The skin covers and protects other body organs, such as bones and muscles. Bones support

TABLE 1.—CLASSIFICATION OF TISSUES

Epithelial Tissue
{
1. Surface cells of covering and of lining membranes (as of skin and of mucous membranes)
2. Glandular tissue
}

Connective Tissue
{
1. Fibrous (as in skin beneath the epithelium)
2. Loose areolar (as in thin membranes between various layers of tissue)
3. Adipose (fat)
4. Hemopoietic (= blood-forming: bone marrow, lymphatic tissue)
5. Cartilage
6. Bone
}

Nerve Tissue
{
1. Tissue of central nervous system
2. Tissue of peripheral nervous system
}

Muscle Tissue
{
1. Smooth involuntary (as in wall of intestines)
2. Striated voluntary (as in skeletal muscle)
3. Striated involuntary (heart muscle)
}

the body, and muscles move the bones and other organs under the direction of the nervous system which supplies the impulses. The entire organism is nourished by blood pumped through the pipe line of the blood vessels by the cardiac muscle, which is the chief tissue of the heart.

EPITHELIAL TISSUE

Epithelial tissue is distributed widely throughout the body and has many different kinds of structure. It occurs as a covering or a lining tissue making up both the surface layer of the skin and the surface layer of the mucous membranes which line body cavities such as the mouth, the stomach, and the intestines. Epithelial tissue also gives rise to several organs during embryonic development. Of epithelial origin in the developing embryo are the highly specialized cells of such organs as the pancreas, the liver, the thyroid gland, and the salivary glands. Also in certain locations in the upper and lower jaws epithelial tissue becomes differentiated into structures called the *enamel organs* which, located deep in the jaw, produce the enamel on the crowns of developing teeth (Chapter 11).

The various kinds of epithelial tissues are similar to one another in that they have a proportionally large number of cells and very little intercellular substance. They are dissimilar in many ways, their structure in different locations in the body being fortunately adapted to the functions which they perform.

For purposes of description histologists have classified epithelial tissues into two major groups and several subgroups:

1. Surface cells of covering and lining membranes

a. Simple
{
Squamous
Cuboidal
Columnar
}

     b. Pseudostratified columnar

     c. Stratified $\begin{cases} \text{Squamous} \\ \text{Cuboidal} \\ \text{Columnar} \\ \text{Transitional} \end{cases}$

  2. Glandular Tissue

     a. Endocrine glands, *e.g.*, thyroid
     b. Exocrine glands, *e.g.*, salivary glands
     c. Mixed endocrine and exocrine, *e.g.*, liver, pancreas

All types of epithelium will not be discussed here. The enamel organ, which is neither a covering nor a lining membrane nor, in the usual sense, a gland, will be considered in the chapter dealing with the development of teeth. The salivary glands will be described in the chapter on the oral mucous membrane and the salivary glands. The endocrine glands, while important physiologically to the development and health of the structures of the oral cavity, are of little importance in our present study so far as their histologic composition is concerned. These glands will not, therefore, be discussed in this book. The types of epithelium which make up the surface cells of covering and lining membranes will be considered briefly.

Epithelial cells of covering and lining membranes are not all alike in shape and arrangement. The *shape* of epithelial cells is described by the words squamous, cuboidal, and columnar; and the *arrangement* of epithelial cells is described by the words simple, stratified, and pseudostratified. The word *squamous* means scale-like, or flat; and *squamous epithelial cells* are flat cells. *Cuboidal epithelial cells* are roughly cube-shaped; and *columnar epithelial cells* are tall and narrow. When the arrangement of epithelial cells is in a single layer the tissue is said to be *simple epithelium*. When epithelial cells are arranged in several layers the tissue is called *stratified epithelium* (stratified = in layers). The word *pseudostratified* is applied to an arrangement of columnar epithelial cells in which the cells appear to be stratified but are actually in a single layer (pseudo = false).

All *simple epithelium* is very delicate in structure. Simple epithelium is found only in those areas of the body which are subjected to little or no friction in functional use. *Simple squamous epithelium* (a single layer of flat epithelial cells) is found lining the inside of the walls of blood vessels (Fig. 10*A*). *Simple cuboidal epithelium* (a single layer of cuboidal epithelial cells) is found in the covering epithelium of the ovary (Fig. 10*B*). *Simple columnar epithelium* (a single layer of columnar epithelial cells) lines the cervix of the uterus (Fig. 10*C*).

Pseudostratified columnar epithelium (Fig. 10*D*) makes up the epithelial part of the mucous membrane which lines the upper respiratory tract: the maxillary sinuses, the nasal cavity, and the trachea. This epithelium is actually composed of a single layer of columnar epithelial cells; but because in some of the cells the nucleus is located near the base of the cell, while in other cells the nucleus is located nearer the outer end, this epithelium has the appearance of being made up of two or three layers of cells. In the upper respiratory tract the pseudostratified columnar epithelium is supplied with *cilia* and with

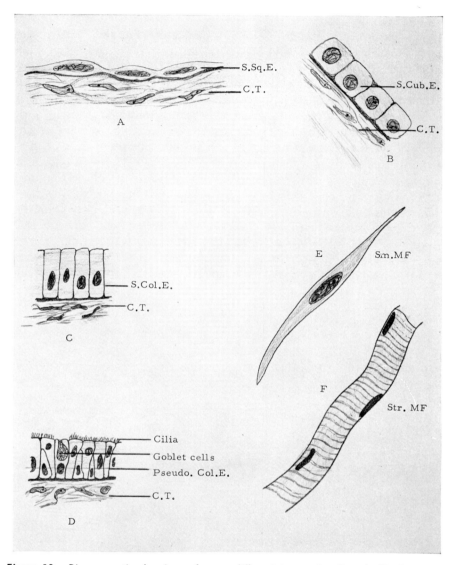

Figure 10. Diagrammatic drawings of some different types of cells.   A. Simple squamous epithelium (S. Sq. E.) resting on connective tissue (C.T.).   B. Simple cuboidal epithelium (S. Cub. E.) resting on connective tissue (C.T.).   C. Simple columnar epithelium (S. Col. E.) resting on connective tissue (C.T).   D. Pseudostratified columnar epithelium (Pseudo. Col. E.) resting on connective tissue (C.T.).   E. A smooth muscle fiber.   F. A striated muscle fiber.

goblet cells (Fig. 10D).   Cilia are minute, hair-like projections which cover the surface ends of the columnar cells and act as dust catchers, or filters, for the air breathed in through the nose.   Goblet cells are modified epithelial cells which are interspersed among the other columnar cells and which secrete substances that keep the tissue surface of the nose and sinuses moist.

Stratified epithelium consists of cells which are similar in shape to cells of simple epithelium, but which are arranged so that they are from 2 or 3 to many layers deep.   *Stratified cuboidal epithelium* and *stratified columnar epithelium* occur as the lining of some of the larger ducts of glands, such as the large ducts of the major salivary glands. The stratified epithelial cells which line the urinary bladder change in shape from round to flat, depending on whether the bladder is empty or full, and this epithelium is therefore described as *stratified transitional epithelium*. Stratified epithelium is more resistant to hard use than the simple types of epithelium. By far the most sturdy of all kinds of epithelia is *stratified squamous epithelium* which is found covering all surfaces of the body which are routinely subjected to considerable wear and tear.

Stratified squamous epithelium (Fig. 11) makes up both the surface of the skin and the surface of the mucous membrane of the oral cavity. In both of these locations the epithelium is composed of many layers of cells. The deepest layer of these epithelial cells rests on a fine structure called the *basement membrane* which separates the epithelial tissue from its underlying connective tissue. The epithelial cells of the deepest layer, called *basal cells*, are not flat in shape but are somewhat cuboidal and often show cell division. As these basal cells multiply, some cells are gradually moved toward the outside surface, becoming flatter as they approach the surface and finally becoming

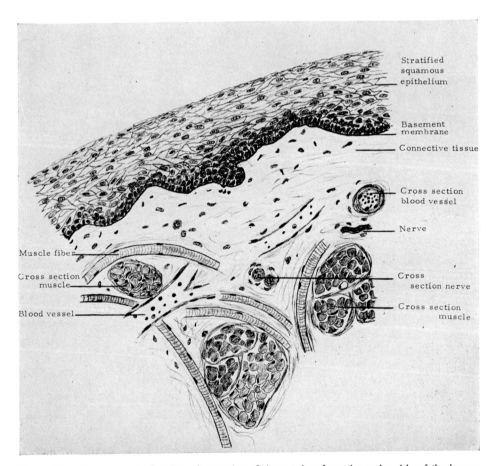

Figure 11. Diagrammatic drawing of a section of tissue taken from the under side of the human tongue. This section illustrates the way in which tissues are combined.

dead cells. In some areas of the oral cavity the flat, dead epithelial cells on the surface are sloughed off as they are replaced from below. In other areas of the oral cavity, and on the skin, these dead surface cells are not quickly sloughed off. Instead they lose their nuclei and their cell boundaries and become converted into a very tough, resistant surface layer which is called the *keratinized layer* (Fig. 77). This keratinized layer, of course, gradually wears off and is replaced from beneath as a result of continued cell division in the basal cell layer. The most heavily keratinized epithelium of the body is found on the palms of the hands and on the soles of the feet, particularly if these areas have been subjected to hard use and are calloused. More about nonkeratinized and keratinzed epithelium will be learned in the study of the oral mucosa.

Covering and lining epithelial tissue does not contain blood vessels; it receives its nourishment via the blood vessels contained in the connective tissue which surrounds or underlies it.

Connective Tissue

The tissues which have been classified together as connective tissue differ from epithelial tissues basically in that they are made up of a relatively larger amount of intercellular substance and relatively fewer cells. In spite of this characteristic which connective tissues have in common they differ so greatly in form and in function that at first glance they sometimes appear to be unrelated. Connective tissue (fibrous) underlies the epithelium of the skin and the epithelium of the oral mucosa and also makes up tendons and ligaments. Connective tissue (areolar) attaches skin to muscle. Connective tissue (fat) stores food. Connective tissue (hemopoietic) forms blood. Connective tissue (cartilage) gives support and permits skeletal growth. Connective tissue (bone) supports the body.

Fibrous connective tissue is found throughout the body. In its most dense form it makes up tendons and ligaments. In a less dense form it is the connective tissue which underlies the epithelial part of skin and of mucous membranes (Figs. 11 and 77). Like other tissues, fibrous connective tissue is made up of cells and intercellular substance, and the intercellular substance is of two kinds: fibrillar and amorphous. The fibrillar component of the intercellular substance is the predominant element.

The fibers of fibrous connective tissue are probably produced by the cells of the tissue which are called *fibroblasts* (blast = germ, builder). The individual fibers are made up of minute fibrils. Special staining techniques used on histologic sections reveal that the fibers are not all alike, some being *collagenous fibers* and others *elastic fibers*. These two types of fibers are distributed in different proportions in different kinds of fibrous connective tissue.

Suspended along with the fibers in the all-encompassing amorphous substance are the various kinds of cells of the fibrous connective tissue. Proportionally the most numerous type of cell is the *fibroblast*. Special tissue preparation will show also the presence of other types of cells, some of which are capable of becoming defense cells when the tissue suffers injury or bacterial infection.

Areolar connective tissue is seen during any gross dissection of a mammal where skin is attached to muscles, muscles to muscles, or where internal organs are held together by membranes of connective tissue. These tissue membranes, called *fascia*, are made up of areolar connective tissue and fat tissue. The areolar connective tissue is composed of a relatively small number of cells and of a very loose and thin network of fibrous intercellular substance, all held together by a large amount of amorphous intercellular substance.

Fat tissue is distributed throughout the body among the soft tissues and in the marrow cavities of bones, and is found more or less generously concentrated in certain parts of the body beneath the skin. It is composed of specialized connective tissue cells, called *fat cells*, which are held together by fibrous intercellular substance. Fat cells are capable of storing fat. They may become so filled with fat that the cytoplasm is pressed into a thin layer around the periphery of the cell, and the nucleus is crowded against the side of the cell.

Hemopoietic tissue (hemo = blood; poietic = to make) not only produces blood cells which are added to the circulating blood, but removes worn out blood cells from the blood stream. In the adult, hemopoietic tissue occurs in two different forms: as *red bone marrow* and as *lymphatic tissue*. In the human fetus, red bone marrow is found in nearly all of the bones; but in the adult, the marrow in many of the bones has become transformed into so-called *yellow bone marrow* (Fig. 76) which is largely fat. Certain bones, however, such as the vault of the skull, the ribs, the sternum, the bodies of vertebrae, retain the red bone marrow throughout adult life. Yellow bone marrow in other bones can be converted into hemopoietic red marrow in circumstances of emergency.

Red bone marrow consists of a fibrillar meshwork of intercellular substance throughout which are scattered many cells which have the potentiality of differentiating into several kinds of blood cells. Red bone marrow produces *red blood cells* and also certain kinds of white blood cells called *granular leukocytes* which are white blood cells that have granules in the cytoplasm (basophils, neutrophils, eosinophils).

Lymphatic tissue is composed of fibrillar intercellular substance and scattered undifferentiated cells. Some of these undifferentiated cells are capable of becoming differentiated into certain kinds of white blood cells, chiefly *lymphocytes*. Conspicuous areas of lymphatic tissue are seen in several places around the oral cavity: the palatine tonsils, which are located between the oral cavity and the pharynx; the pharyngeal tonsils, which are located on the posterior wall of the pharynx; and the lingual tonsils, which are located on the posterior part of the dorsum of the tongue. Lymphatic tissue is found also in other parts of the body.

In *cartilage* the most conspicuous component of the tissue is the amorphous intercellular substance, which in gross examination resembles a firm gel. Fibers, which may be made visible by special histologic preparation of tissue sections, are scattered throughout the amorphous intercellular substance. The cells of cartilage, called *chondrocytes*, occupy spaces, called *lacunae*, in the intercellular substance. Nutrients are transmitted to the cells through the intercellular substance. Cartilage exists as a noncalcified tissue.

A large part of the skeleton of the human fetus is first constructed in cartilage, which seems to act as a pattern for the developing bone tissue. The arm and leg bones, for example, are first formed in cartilage, which is resorbed as bone tissue develops to replace it. While bone replaces most cartilage in the human skeleton at an early stage, cartilage persists in some places for years. At the ends of the long bones the presence of cartilage throughout childhood and adolescence permits growth in the length of the bones. In adults cartilage comprises parts of the nose, larynx, trachea, and ear. Cartilage tissue contains no nerves or blood vessels.

Bone is a calcified connective tissue (Fig. 68). Bone contains a large amount of dense fibrous intercellular substance. The fibrils which make up the fibrous intercellular substance are of course surrounded by amorphous intercellular substance. In the amorphous substance mineral salts are deposited in solution as the bone is developing. As the bone matures, these mineral salts crystallize out of solution and the bone becomes a calcified tissue. The cells of bone, called *osteocytes*, occupy spaces known as *lacunae* in the hard intercellular substance. More will be learned in a later chapter about the microscopic picture of bone tissue.

NERVE TISSUE

Nerve tissue, which comprises the total nervous system, is made up of nerve cells and a tissue which supports them. Nerve cells are called *neurons* and they are like other cells in that they have a nucleus and a cytoplasm. However, they are highly specialized, that is, different from other cells, in that they have to a high degree the properties of reacting to stimuli (irritability) and of transmitting waves of excitation from the point where the stimulus is applied (conductivity). These waves of excitation, or *nerve impulses* as they are called, are transmitted through the cytoplasm of the neuron which is peculiarly adapted to this function.

The nervous system consists of two chief divisions: the *central nervous system* (the brain and spinal cord) and the *peripheral nervous system* (nerves associated with the various other organs of the body). The gross appearance and the histologic structure of the nerve tissue in these two divisions are very different. The tissue of the central nervous system is extremely soft due to the absence of connective tissue as a supporting tissue for the nerve cells. In the central nervous system the nerve cells are supported by a delicate and very fragile tissue called *neuroglia* (literally, nerve glue). The brain and spinal cord are made up of two distinct types of this soft nerve tissue called *gray matter* and *white matter* which differ greatly in histologic structure.

In contrast to the nerve tissue of the central nervous system the nerves of the peripheral nervous system are tough. This firm quality is derived from the considerable amount of connective tissue which covers and supports the bundles of nerve fibers. A microscopic examination of a cross section of a nerve shows it to be circular in shape and covered by a connective tissue wrapping, or *sheath*. Inside this sheath are several bundles of *nerve fibers*, each bundle being surrounded by another connective tissue sheath. Each nerve fiber inside the bundles is encased in its individual connective tissue sheath, and often between this sheath and the individual fiber is a layer of substance of a fatty nature called a *myelin sheath*. Each nerve fiber in this nerve is actually a long, thin, stretched-out part of the cytoplasm of a neuron. The body of the neuron, which contains the nucleus, lies deep in the body of the individual.

Nerve cells do not multiply with the growth of the human body. A person is born with all the neurons he will ever possess. However, if a fiber in the peripheral nervous system is cut, repair may eventually take place. The end of the fiber which has been cut off from the body of the neuron will degenerate, and the end of the fiber still attached to the neuron may after a time grow out to the length of the original fiber. In the central nervous system, on the other hand, damage is permanent. There is no regeneration following damage to the brain or spinal cord.

MUSCLE TISSUE

Muscle tissue is composed of muscle cells which are supported by connective tissue. Muscle cells are in all cases much longer than they are wide, and for this reason an individual muscle cell is called a muscle fiber. Muscle fibers have to a greater degree than other cells the property of contraction.

Microscopic examination of muscle tissue from various parts of the body shows a difference in the appearance of the cytoplasm of muscle fibers. In muscle tissue from some areas, for example from the intestine, the cytoplasm of the muscle fibers appears relatively clear. In muscle tissue from other areas, such as from the arm or the heart, the cytoplasm of the muscle fibers has conspicuous cross striations. This difference in the appearance of the cytoplasm of different muscle fibers led histologists to classify muscle tissue as *smooth muscle tissue* (where the cytoplasm of the fibers is not cross striated), and *striated muscle tissue* (where the cytoplasm of the fibers is cross striated). (See Figure 10E and F.)

This division of muscle tissue into two types was not quite adequate, however. Smooth muscle is *involuntary muscle*—that is, the contraction of its fibers is not under the control of the will of the individual. For instance, the peristaltic movements of the intestine, which contains smooth muscle in its walls, are not willfully controlled. On the other hand, striated muscle is for the most part *voluntary muscle* because the contractions of the muscle fibers may be consciously controlled by the individual. One moves an arm or a leg as one wishes. However, there is an exception. The fibers of heart muscle, although striated like the fibers of the muscles of the arm, are not consciously controlled by the individual. Therefore cardiac muscle has been described as belonging to a class by itself and is called *striated involuntary muscle* in contrast to skeletal muscle which is referred to as *striated voluntary muscle*.

Thus we arrive at a classification for muscle tissue consisting of three categories: *smooth muscle, striated voluntary muscle*, and *striated involuntary muscle*.

Smooth muscle tissue is found in such places as in the walls of the intestines, in the walls of blood vessels, and at the roots of hairs where its contraction produces an erection of the hair. The individual muscle fibers (cells) of smooth muscle tissue are shaped somewhat like a cigar and have a centrally located nucleus (Fig. 10E). In length they may vary from 1/1000 mm. in the small blood vessels to $\frac{1}{2}$ mm. in the pregnant uterus. The fibers are supported by associated connective tissue.

Striated voluntary muscle is known also as *skeletal muscle*. As well as the obvious inclusion in this class of such muscles as those which move the arms and legs, skeletal muscles also include those in and about the oral cavity: muscles of the tongue, of the lips and cheeks, of the soft palate. The muscle fibers of skeletal muscle differ in a number of ways from those of smooth muscle. Most conspicuous of course is the difference in the appearance of the cytoplasm, which shows microscopic cross striations (Fig. 10F). Also, the nuclei in skeletal muscle fibers are pushed to one side of the fibers instead of lying in the center, and there is more than one nucleus in a fiber. Skeletal muscle fibers are relatively long, varying from 1 to 40 mm., and they are supported by connective tissue which not only covers individual fibers, but binds the fibers into bundles. This supporting connective tissue is well supplied with blood vessels and nerves.

Striated involuntary muscle is confined to the heart and is known also as *cardiac muscle*. In microscopic appearance it resembles skeletal muscle in that the cytoplasm of the muscle fibers has microscopic cross striations. Its appearance differs from that of skeletal muscle in the arrangement of the fibers. Whereas skeletal muscle fibers exist as individual fibers with several nuclei, cardiac muscle fibers branch and come together so that they form a sort of network which comprises the heart muscle. This network is supported by surrounding connective tissue which contains nerves and a rich supply of blood vessels.

Muscles are the organs responsible for both the voluntary and the involuntary movement of all of the various parts of the body. They act in response to impulses received from the nervous system. They are surrounded by, supported by, and nourished by the different kinds of connective tissue: the fibrous areolar, and adipose; the bone and cartilage; and the blood.

ORAL HISTOLOGY

Of particular importance in Dentistry are the tissues of the oral cavity. The entire practice of Dentistry and Dental Hygiene is based on a knowledge of the structure, arrangement, and reactions of oral tissues. Instructions given to a patient by the dentist and the dental hygienist concerning the correct method of brushing the teeth are based on a knowledge of oral histology. A dentist prepares a tooth for a filling with careful attention to the nature and arrangement of the tissues comprising the tooth; and he constructs an artificial denture with regard for the structure of the tissues of the palate, of the alveolar ridge, and of the oral vestibule. The pathosis which occurs in the tissues around a tooth when calculus is present can be understood only in the light of a knowledge of tissue structure and tissue reaction; and the tissue repair which follows removal of the calculus is explainable in the same terms. Other diseases of the soft tissues of the mouth are recognized and treated only as normal tissue structure is known. The nearly universal disease of the hard tooth tissues, dental caries, must be described in terms of the microscopic structure of the calcified tissues of a tooth.

Oral histology is the study of the tissues of the oral cavity: the tissues lining the mouth and the tissues beneath the lining, the tissues of the tongue, the periodontium, the tooth, and the tissues from which a tooth develops. This book will include also a study of the process of tooth development.

LOCATION OF ORAL TISSUES

The relative locations of some of the oral tissues may be seen in the diagram of a section through a human mandible in the region of the second premolar tooth (Fig. 66). The *tooth* is attached by fibers of the *periodontal ligament* to the *lamina dura* which comprises the tooth socket. The outside surface of the mandible consists of *cortical plate* inside of which is *trabecular bone* and bone marrow. The lining of the inside of the cheek, the gingiva, and the covering of the *tongue* are mucous membrane. Under the tongue are located the *salivary glands* and several *muscles*.

TISSUES OF A TOOTH

The tissues which make up a tooth are the enamel, the dentin, the cementum, and the pulp. Figures 12, 13, 14 and 15 are diagrams of teeth which have been cut approximately through the middle in a faciolingual direction. *Tooth enamel* comprises the surface of the crown of the tooth and *cementum* comprises the surface of the tooth root. *Dentin*, which lies beneath the enamel of the crown and beneath the cementum of the root, makes up the bulk of the hard tissue of the tooth. The *tooth pulp* is the only noncalcified tissue of the tooth. It occupies the *pulp chamber* in the crown of the tooth and continues through the *root canals* to its union with the periodontal ligament at the *apical foramen*.

The line of union between the dentin and the enamel is the *dentinoenamel junction*. The line of union between the dentin and the cementum is the *dentinocemental junction*. The line of union between the cementum and the enamel is the *cementoenamel junction*. These are frequent points of reference in descriptions of a tooth.

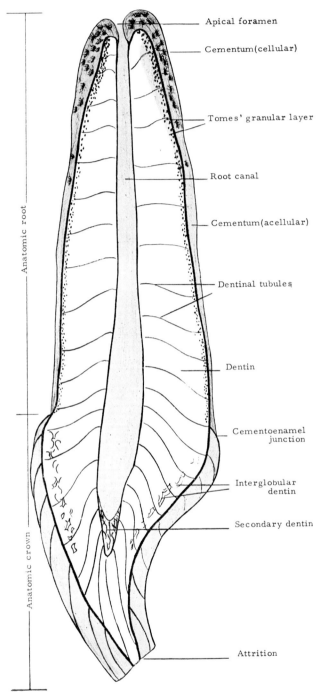

Figure 12. Diagrammatic drawing of a longitudinal faciolingual section of a maxillary incisor tooth. The cementum lacunae in this and in the following diagrams of tooth sections are somewhat exaggerated in size. For identification of unlabeled structures see Figures 13, 14 and 15.

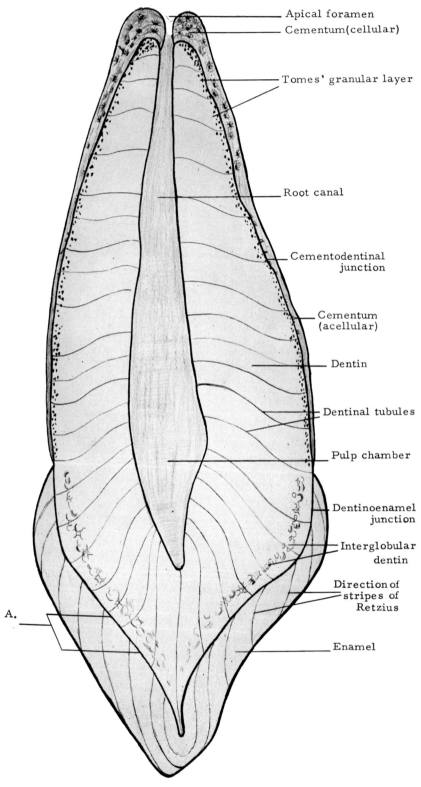

Apical foramen

Cementum(cellular)

Tomes' granular layer

Root canal

Cementodentinal junction

Cementum (acellular)

Dentin

Dentinal tubules

Pulp chamber

Dentinoenamel junction

Interglobular dentin

Direction of stripes of Retzius

A.

Enamel

Figure 13. Diagrammatic drawing of a longitudinal faciolingual section of a maxillary canine tooth. The area marked *A* indicates a location in the enamel similar to that shown in Figure 25.

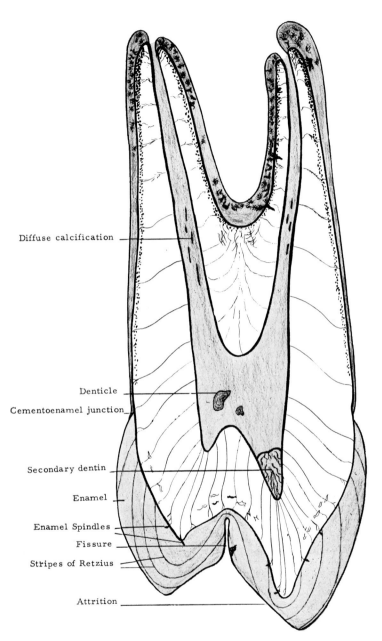

Diffuse calcification

Denticle

Cementoenamel junction

Secondary dentin

Enamel

Enamel Spindles

Fissure

Stripes of Retzius

Attrition

Figure 14. Diagrammatic drawing of a longitudinal faciolingual section of a maxillary first premolar tooth. See Figure 1 for a photograph of a similar tooth and compare the structures indicated in the diagrammatic drawing with the same structures seen in the photograph of the actual tooth section.

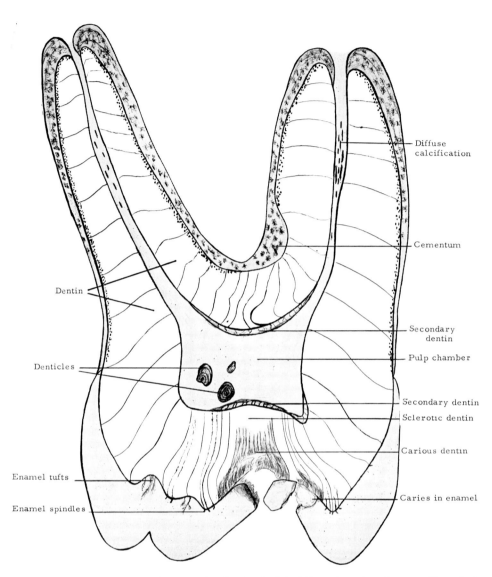

Figure 15. Diagrammatic drawing of a longitudinal faciolingual section of a maxillary first molar tooth. Dental caries has destroyed the enamel in the area around a developmental groove on the occlusal surface. The caries has spread horizontally at the dentinoenamel junction, with a resultant undermining of enamel. Caries has spread pulpward in the dentinal tubules to about $\frac{2}{3}$ the thickness of the dentin. The dentin close to the pulp is sclerotic dentin: the tubules are filled with mineral salts. On the pulpal wall beneath the caries lesion a small amount of secondary dentin has formed. The secondary dentin on the floor of the pulp chamber (next to the root) was not caused by caries; secondary dentin in this location is not unusual. (See Figure 39.)

CHAPTER 3

Tooth Enamel

LOCATION

Tooth enamel makes up the outside layer of the anatomic crown of a tooth (Figs. 1 and 12).

COMPOSITION

Enamel is composed of both inorganic (mineral) and organic substances. Mature human enamel is about 96 per cent inorganic. The remaining 4 per cent of its substance is an organic matrix (framework) and water. Enamel is the hardest tissue of the body, its mineral content far exceeding the mineral content of dentin (70 per cent), of cementum (50 per cent), or of bone (50 per cent).

MACROSCOPIC STRUCTURE OF ENAMEL

Examine the teeth of several persons who maintain reasonably good oral hygiene. The crown surfaces are composed of hard, shiny enamel. In young individuals who are free from dental caries, no other tooth tissues are exposed in the oral cavity. On some of the teeth of older individuals, due to a normal aging process, the gingiva may have receded to such an extent that cementum is visible. In persons of any age whose teeth have unrepaired caries lesions, dentin will be exposed in the areas where the disease has destroyed the enamel.

On the labial surfaces of the maxillary central incisors of a young person you usually see a number of fine horizontal lines on the enamel. In the cervical part of the crown these lines are close together; incisally on the crown they are farther apart (Fig. 16). These lines are called *perikymata*.* Their presence is not confined to the maxillary central incisors; they are found on the enamel of all surfaces of all teeth, but they are easier to see on the more accessible surfaces. In older persons perikymata usually are not visible.

Examination of the teeth of persons of different ages will show that generally in older persons the enamel appears darker in color than in younger persons. The reason for this darkening is not clearly understood.

Despite its hardness tooth enamel is subject to *attrition*—that is, wearing off under the friction of use. Examine the teeth of several middle-aged persons. Probably you will find the enamel of the molar cusps worn so that the cusp tips are nearly flat. Sometimes the enamel is entirely worn off of the

* Pronounced *pĕr ĭ kī' mȧt ȧh*.

Figure 16. Labial surface of a maxillary central incisor tooth.
The horizontal lines are perikymata.

cusp tips and the exposed dentin is seen as dark spots (Fig. 17). In the anterior teeth the incisal edges of the central and lateral incisors may be sufficiently worn so that dentin is seen as a fine dark line extending mesiodistally on the incisal edge (Fig. 28). These conditions of attrition in older individuals are not abnormal but are merely a natural aging process. Accompanying changes in the dentin beneath the worn enamel protect the tooth pulp from damage (Chapter 4, sclerotic and secondary dentin).

Examine the newly emerged incisor teeth of a six- or seven-year-old child. There are probably three prominences, or scallops, along the incisal edge. These prominences are called *mamelons*.* They are developmental structures, but are ordinarily of no clinical importance. Usually they are worn off early in the life of the tooth. (Figs. 38 and 61).

In an adult mouth look carefully at the posterior teeth and observe the developmental grooves that mark the occlusal surfaces. Developmental grooves will also be found on the buccal surfaces of maxillary and mandibular molars (Fig. 111), on the lingual surfaces of maxillary molars, and sometimes on the lingual surfaces of maxillary incisors. The structure of developmental grooves varies: In some teeth they are shallow and smooth (Figs. 29 and 30) while in others they are extended into deep fissures (Figs. 1, 21, 31, 32, 33). On occlusal surfaces the grooves and fissures may end in

* Pronounced *măm' ĕl ons.*

deep pits in the mesial and distal triangular fossae or in the central fossa. On the buccal and lingual surfaces the grooves may have a deep pit at their cervical end. It will be impossible to see, in examining the mouth, how deep such fissures and pits are; and usually it will be impossible to insert even the smallest dental instrument or toothbrush bristle into them (Figs. 1 and 21). The pit or fissure does not extend into the dentin; it always ends in the enamel. And there is always a little enamel, however thin, at the base of the pit or fissure (Figs. 21, 31, 32, 33). Enamel structure in fissures is studied, of course, not by looking in the mouth, but by examination of ground sections of extracted teeth.

In thickness the enamel varies in different parts of the tooth crown. At its thickest parts it may be 2 or 2.5 mm. thick, while at the cervical line it thins to a knife edge. Examine Figures 12, 13, 14, 15 and 18 for an idea of the relative thickness of the enamel in different locations.

Enveloping the crown of the tooth, and adhering firmly to its surface, is the *enamel cuticle*, a layer of material which has been the subject of many studies since it was first described by Alexander Nasmyth in 1842. Early histologists called it *Nasmyth's membrane*, and this name is still widely used.

Through the years this crown covering has been described in ways so diverse that it seems certain that not one, but several substances were being observed. At different times it has been said to consist of cementum, of denatured hemoglobin, and of substances from saliva. The nature of what Nasmyth saw is not clear, and probably it would be better to refer to the covering, whatever it is, not as Nasmyth's membrane, but as *enamel cuticle*.

Figure 17. Attrition has almost exposed the dentin on the two buccal and two lingual cusps of this mandibular first molar. There is no apparent attrition on the distal cusp. Notice the developmental pits at the cervical end of both the mesial and distal buccal grooves.

Undoubtedly, in time the electron microscope will give a clear picture of what covers the enamel of unerupted and erupted teeth. So far, studies of electron micrographs have not led to consistent interpretations. Therefore, for practical purposes, enamel cuticle will be described in the traditional manner.

Enamel cuticle is actually two cuticles: *primary enamel cuticle* and *secondary enamel cuticle*. The primary enamel cuticle is the last product of the enamel-forming cells (*ameloblasts*, described in Chapter 11), and it becomes calcified. Secondary enamel cuticle is a product of the reduced enamel epithelium (Chapter 11), and it does not become calcified. The secondary enamel cuticle is the outermost layer and it probably wears away after a period of tooth use.

Microscopic Structure of Enamel

Enamel can be studied by various methods. With an ordinary microscope you can examine thin ground sections of extracted teeth and see in their natural relationship the organic and inorganic substances which comprise enamel. Or the organic portion, the matrix, which is in the form of a delicate framework, can be examined separately by using special careful techniques to dissolve away the mineral substances. In recent years new techniques have enabled the histologist to study enamel and other tooth tissues with the electron microscope at magnifications of the order of 5,000 × to 40,000 × and more.

Tooth enamel is made up of minute *rods** which extend from the dentino-enamel junction to the outer surface of the enamel. They are arranged roughly perpendicular to the dentinoenamel junction (Fig. 18). Seldom are the rods perfectly straight; in some parts of the tooth they have multiple curvatures. It has been estimated that a human maxillary central incisor contains 8,586,000 enamel rods, and that a maxillary first molar contains 12,297,000 rods. The average diameter of a rod is about 4 microns ($\frac{4}{1000}$ millimeter). Each enamel rod is composed of a series of small units which fit together in a row somewhat like a string of beads (Figs. 19 and 42). This segmented construction is a result of the manner of formation of the enamel rods (Chapter 11).

Each enamel rod is encased in a *rod sheath*, and the sheathed rods are cemented together by an *interrod substance*. Of these three structures, the rods are the most highly calcified, the cementing substance is slightly less calcified than the rods, and the rod sheaths are slightly less calcified than the cementing substance. However, all three structures are extremely hard. The organic substance which they contain has been shown by the electron microscope to be in the form of a fine fibrillar latticework. This latticework, or framework, of the rods, rod sheaths, and interrod substance is the *organic matrix* of the enamel. In suitable preparations this matrix may be examined with an ordinary microscope, but the fibrils of which it is composed are so minute that its fibrillar character can be seen only by the use of the electron microscope.

The entire organic substance of enamel comprises only about 4 per cent of its composition. The other 96 per cent of enamel is mineral substance

* Another name for an *enamel rod* is *enamel prism*.

Figure 18. Diagrammatic drawing of a longitudinal faciolingual section of the crown of a maxillary first premolar tooth. The lines in the enamel illustrate the general direction of the enamel rods. Notice the narrowness of the fissure (F) and the thinness of the enamel at the bottom of the fissure. Notice also the radiating pattern of the enamel rods in the fissure.

Figure 19. A photomicrograph (high power) of a ground section of human enamel showing the rods extending from the dentinoenamel junction to the tooth surface. The rods extend from top to bottom of the picture and in this area they are nearly straight. The cross striations in the rods are discernible.

which exists in the form of tightly packed *submicroscopic crystals*. These crystals fill the loose organic matrix. Their size is appreciated when we learn that they are measured in terms of millionths of a millimeter.

To the best of our knowledge today, this description of enamel is essentially true. But as in every age back into antiquity, current ideas are constantly challenged, and as a result of man's compelling search for knowledge some "truths" stand and others fall.

Electron microscope studies since 1944 have confirmed many of the conclusions concerning tooth structure reached by earlier observers with ordinary microscopes. However, some established ideas have been opened to doubt, and others are seriously questioned. For instance, some investigators believe that there exists no actual rod sheath and interrod substance. Instead, they explain the appearance of what seems to be these structures as due to differences in orientation of the submicroscopic crystals in areas around the rods. Also, doubt has been cast on the shape of the enamel rods. In cross section the rods in some enamel appear to be the shape of a keyhole or even of a horseshoe, instead of roughly hexagonal as has been thought. However, these apparent variations in shape may sometimes, or possibly always, be determined by the angle at which the specimen is cut. These questions, and many others, are the focus of much study, and the findings are at present subject to diverse interpretations. Interpretations that seem correct today, tomorrow may be doubted.

In Figure 20 the electron micrograph of a replica of human enamel reveals rod outlines. Most of the submicroscopic crystals have been dissolved by the acid-etching which was part of the process of preparation of the specimen. What is seen in the picture is interpreted to be the organic matrix of the enamel.

Electron microscopy is immensely important, because when the pieces of the puzzle are better assembled our knowledge of tooth structure will be immeasurably extended. The student interested in learning more in this field should have the pleasure and satisfaction of starting with a recently published paper and, following its bibliography, tracing the development of the subject back to its beginning.*

Examination with an ordinary microscope of a thin ground tooth section reveals other structures in enamel: *bands of Hunter-Schreger, stripes of Retzius, enamel lamellae, enamel tufts,* and *enamel spindles.* Some of these structures are of little known clinical importance, while others are of great importance.

Bands of Hunter-Schreger are seen when a longitudinal ground section of a tooth crown is examined by reflected light under the low power of the micro-

---

* Interesting papers:
1. Hoffman, S., W. S. McEwan, and C. M. Drew: Scanning Electron Microscope Studies of Dental Enamel, Jour. Dent. Res. *48*:242, 1969.
2. Meckel, A. H., W. J. Griebstein, and R. J. Neal: Structure of Mature Human Dental Enamel as Observed by Electron Microscopy, Arch. Oral Biol. *10*:775, 1965.
3. Poole, D. F. G. and N. W. Johnson: Effects of Different Demineralizing Agents on Human Enamel Surfaces Studied by the Scanning Electron Microscope, Arch. Oral Biol. *12*:1621, 1967.
4. Johnson, N. W., D. F. Poole, and J. E. Tyler: Factors Affecting the Differential Dissolution of Human Enamel in Acid and EDTA, Arch. Oral Biol. *16*:385, 1971.

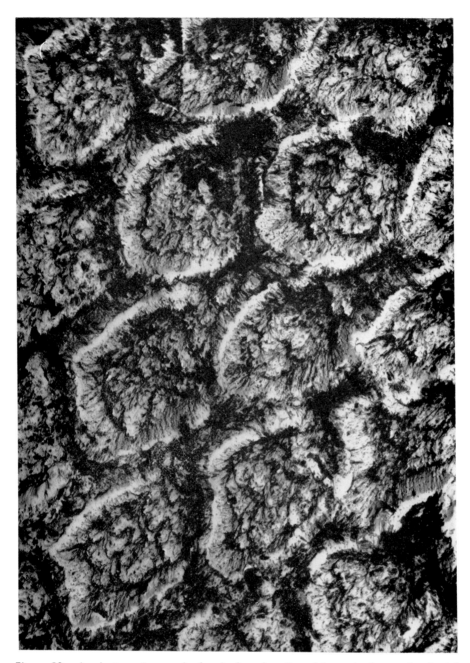

Figure 20. An electron micrograph of a shadowed replica of the ends of enamel rods at the buccal surface of a mature human incisor. The clean enamel surface was first lightly acid-etched; then a nitrocellulose film in a softened state was placed over the etched surface. When the dried film was removed, it of course carried the image of the etched surface. This film, called the *replica*, was shadowed at an angle of 40° with a palladium and gold alloy which gave it contrast and a third dimensional character by creating lights and shadows. The original magnification of the electron micrograph of the shadowed replica was 3,400 ×.

What is seen here is interpreted to be the organic matrix of the enamel; most of the mineral substance was removed by the earlier acid-etching. The rods are seen in end view, but there is no way of knowing how near to an *exact* cross section of the rods we are seeing. The broad white band around each rod conforms to what is considered the rod sheath, and the substance between the rods is interpreted as the interrod substance. (Courtesy Dr. Dennis Foreman, College of Dentistry, The Ohio State University.)

scope (Fig. 21). They are alternating broad light and dark bands which extend perpendicularly from the dentinoenamel junction to the tooth surface. Their manifestation is due to the curvature of the enamel rods.

The *stripes of Retzius* are a different kind of bands, or lines, in the enamel. In longitudinal ground sections of the tooth crown they are seen under the low power of the microscope as narrow brownish lines extending diagonally outward from the dentinoenamel junction toward the occlusal, or incisal, part of the crown (Figs. 13, 14, 21 and 22). These structures are formed during the development of the enamel matrix as a result of the layer-upon-layer pattern of enamel matrix formation. They are due to variations in structure and calcification along the lines corresponding to the formation pattern. On most of the crown the stripes of Retzius end on the crown surface, and their termination on the surface is marked by a series of shallow depressions. The ridges between the depressions are called the *perikymata*. (It is difficult to see in ground tooth sections this association between perikymata and the

Figure 21. Ground section cut buccolingually through a mandibular molar tooth. In the enamel the dark and light bands of Hunter-Schreger extend from the dentinoenamel junction to the enamel surface nearly perpendicular to the dentinoenamel junction. The stripes of Retzius are faintly visible, starting at the dentinoenamel junction and extending outward and occlusally, reaching the enamel surface excepting near the cusp tip (see Fig. 14). In this tooth there is some attrition on the cusp tips. Considering the magnification of this picture, it is clear that the fissure is too narrow to permit the insertion of any dental instrument. The enamel at the bottom of the fissure is thin. It shows no sign of caries.

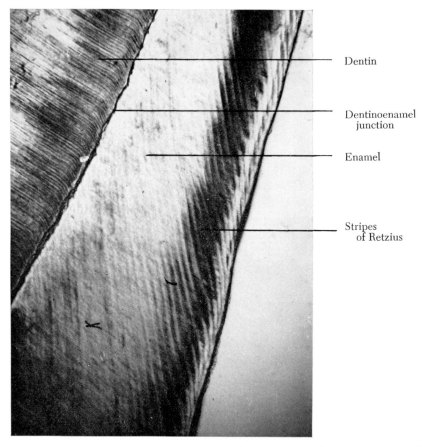

Dentin

Dentinoenamel
junction

Enamel

Stripes
of Retzius

Figure 22. A photomicrograph of a small area of tooth crown cut longitudinally. Stripes of Retzius in the enamel are clearly visible. The direction of the dentinal tubules can also be seen. (Occlusal surface toward bottom of picture; root toward top.)

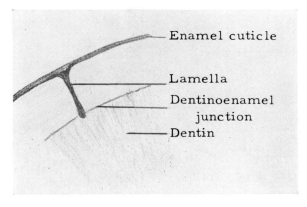

Enamel cuticle

Lamella
Dentinoenamel
junction
Dentin

Figure 23. Schematic diagram of a small area of a cross section of a tooth crown in the region of an enamel lamella.

stripes of Retzius.) Near the incisal or occlusal part of the crown the stripes of Retzius do not reach the enamel surface and therefore there are no perikymata at the incisal edge or cusp tips (Fig. 14). Perikymata often may be seen in clinical examination (Fig. 16).

Enamel lamellae (literally the word means *little layers*) have been described by some histologists as faults in enamel matrix formation and by others as cracks in the enamel due to injury. Certainly they are microscopic separations in the enamel which extend inward from the enamel surface for varying distances and which are filled with organic material (Fig. 23). Lamellae may sometimes be seen by using the low power of the microscope on a ground section of tooth crown.

Enamel tufts also are visible in ground tooth sections. Microscopically they look like small brushes which are attached to the dentinoenamel junction and which extend outward in the enamel to perhaps as much as a fifth of the distance to the surface (Figs. 15 and 24). Histologically they are hypocalcified, or uncalcified, inner ends of some groups of enamel rods, with their rod sheaths and surrounding interrod substance.

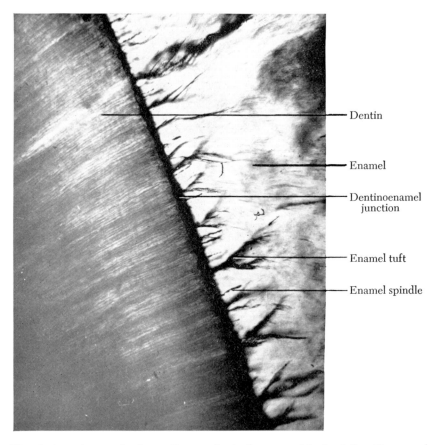

Dentin

Enamel

Dentinoenamel junction

Enamel tuft

Enamel spindle

Figure 24. A photomicrograph of a small area of a tooth crown cut horizontally. The enamel tufts are clearly visible. Among the tufts, in some places, are seen the much smaller enamel spindles. (As seen under low power magnification.)

Enamel spindles are ends of dentinal fibers which project from the dentin across the dentinoenamel junction into the enamel (Figs. 14, 24, 25, 26, 27). These structures will be understood when you study the structure of dentin.

The *dentinoenamel junction* in many teeth is not a straight line, but rather a scalloped line in which small curved projections of enamel fit into small concavities of the dentin (Fig. 42).

Enamel contains no cells; it is a product of special enamel-forming cells. It has no circulation in the form of blood vessels or other structures, but that it is permeable to some substances has been demonstrated in studies using dyes and solutions of radioactive substances. Any clinical significance of this permeability is not at present understood.

Dentin

Dentinal tubule and dentinal fiber

Dentinoenamel junction

Enamel

Enamel spindle

Direction of enamel rods

An enamel rod, showing striations

Figure 25. Diagrammatic drawing of details of area A in Figure 13 showing enamel spindles.

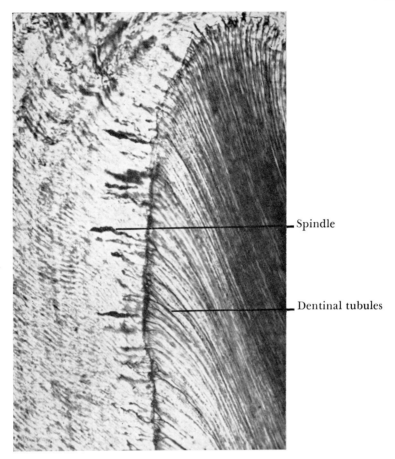

Spindle

Dentinal tubules

Figure 26. A ground section of a tooth crown near cusp tip. Enamel is on left of the picture dentin on right. Many enamel spindles are protruding from the dentinoenamel junction. Notice that the direction of the spindles is different from the direction of the rods of the enamel (medium power magnification.)

Dentinal
tubule

Spindle

Figure 27. Photomicrograph of an enamel spindle as seen with the oil immersion objective of the microscope. Enamel is at left, dentin is at right of the picture. It is possible to see that the spindle was a continuation of the dentinal fiber. Notice the branching of the dentinal tubules at the dentinoenamel junction (Chapter 4).

44

Permanence of Enamel Structure

Once tooth enamel is formed the calcification is never decreased by any physiological process within the tooth. All present evidence indicates that mineral substance is not withdrawn from enamel once it has been deposited there. The notion that pregnancy produces a withdrawal of calcium from the teeth of the mother is not supported by factual evidence.

Enamel has no possibility of anatomic self-repair following damage by injury or by caries. In the study of tooth eruption it will be seen that the cells which form the enamel in the developing tooth are lost when the tooth emerges into the mouth, making subsequent enamel formation impossible.

Clinical Importance of the Structure of Enamel

The structure of enamel is important clinically for several reasons: its hardness makes it resistant to the friction of ordinary use; the curvatures of the enamel rods probably increase the strength of the enamel; the presence of pits and fissures influences the occurrence of dental caries; and the arrangement of the enamel rods and the presence of areas of less mineralization influence the pattern and speed of progress of dental caries.

Let us consider how the structure of enamel may affect the clinical condition of an individual.

The high mineral content of enamel makes it a very hard substance which is resistant to, but not proof against, attrition (Figs. 12, 21, 32 and 74). On the incisal edges of anterior teeth and on the cusp tips of posterior teeth, where the teeth of opposing arches meet forcefully in occlusion, attrition may be sufficient to expose the underlying dentin (Figs. 17 and 28).

Figure 28. An extracted maxillary left central incisor tooth photographed from the incisal aspect. The facial surface is toward the top. Attrition on the incisal edge has exposed the dentin. This edge was not ground off; this is the result of wear from the friction of use. Notice the thickness of the enamel. The caries lesion showing in the dentin on the mesial side (to the left) started on the enamel surface around the mesial contact area. A diagonally placed groove can be seen on the cingulum.

The *perikymata* which usually mark the enamel on all surfaces of all teeth are of no known clinical importance.

The *bands of Hunter-Schreger* are visible in ground sections of teeth. They are due to the curvatures in the enamel rods. These curvatures probably make the enamel stronger by reducing the chances of cleavage (splitting) of the enamel along the rod length.

Enamel lamellae are believed by some investigators to be areas which are particularly susceptible to dental caries. Other investigators disagree.

The *stripes of Retzius*, being areas of slightly less mineral material, tend to facilitate the lateral spread of caries along the line of each stripe. However, this lateral spread is considerably less pronounced than the lateral spread of caries which occurs along the dentinoenamel junction in areas of tufts and spindles.

Enamel tufts and *enamel spindles*, being unmineralized or hypomineralized, offer little resistance to the enlargement of a lesion. The surface enamel may show injury only at the point of initial damage, while beneath this point caries spreads laterally at the dentinoenamel junction (Figs. 33 and 34*B*). When the damaging agent enters dentin, lateral spread of caries is even more extensive (Chapter 4).

To understand the role of tooth structure in the occurrence and pattern of dental caries, it is necessary to understand the nature of this disease. Dental caries is a disease of the hard tissues of the teeth in which the mineral substance of the tooth is dissolved by acid and the then-exposed organic substance is destroyed by proteolysis. The acid is created by the kinds of oral bacteria which, in the process of their metabolism, convert carbohydrates, especially sugars, into acids. Caries-susceptible individuals have in their saliva and in their dental plaques large numbers of these acidogenic (acid-producing) bacteria.

The bacteria which cause the damage are the ones which are located in the dental plaques. A *dental plaque* is a dense accumulation of microorganisms which adheres firmly to the surface of a tooth. In mouths kept ordinarily clean, plaques are found chiefly in protected areas—around contact areas, and in pits and fissures (Fig. 29).

A known sequence of events follows the oral intake of sugar by a caries-susceptible person: Food taken into the mouth is retained in the area of the plaque; the acidogenic bacteria of the plaque reduce the sugars to acids; the acids in the plaque are in contact with the tooth surface to which the plaque is attached; and since tooth enamel is soluble in acid, the enamel beneath the plaque is slightly dissolved. This is the beginning of a caries lesion. Repeated eating of sugar results in repeated periods of enamel dissolution.

PITS AND FISSURES AND CARIES

Particularly prone to caries are the grooves, fissures, and pits of the posterior teeth. While teeth without fissures and pits (Figs. 29 and 30) often—not always—remain intact in their shallow grooves, teeth with fissures and pits have in the depths of these narrow depressions an ideal environment for the growth of microorganisms. Although the fissure or pit may be so narrow

Figure 29. Ground section cut buccolingually through a mandibular first premolar tooth. The developmental groove on the occlusal surface of the tooth is not deep, and there is no fissure at its base. No caries is present in this groove. A plaque is retained in the groove. If the plaque is mineralized, it is called calculus.

Notice the direction of the dentinal tubules which extend from the dentinoenamel junction to the pulp chamber (Chapter 4).

Figure 30. Ground section of a molar tooth. The developmental groove on the occlusal surface does not have a fissure at its base. No dental caries is present in the groove. Notice the direction of the dentinal tubules. The pulp horn extends far into the cusp (Chapter 5).

and so deep that even the smallest instrument cannot be inserted to the bottom (Figs. 21, 31, 32, 33), it still permits the entrance of microorganisms and food into this sheltered, warm, moist, richly provided incubator, and a dental plaque can be expected to form here (Figs. 31 and 32). In a caries-susceptible person, when sugar is eaten and comes in contact with the plaque, acid is created by acidogenic bacteria in the plaque and this acid damages the enamel walls of the pit or fissure. Caries results.

In pit and fissure caries, or in caries occurring around contact areas, or in caries in any other location on the tooth crown, the pattern of arrangement of the enamel rods in the affected area determines the direction of penetration of the lesion. This is true because caries progresses rapidly in areas between the rods. The rod sheaths and the interrod substance seem to be less mineralized than the rods, and in microscopic examination of carious enamel it can be seen that the lesion penetrates through the interrod substance along the direction of the rod length.

On the smooth facial, lingual, and proximal surfaces of a tooth the general direction of the enamel rods is nearly perpendicular to the straight or broadly convex dentinoenamel junction (Fig. 18), even though in many places the rods show characteristic curvatures (seen as the bands of Hunter-Schreger). Therefore, a lesion occurring around a contact area, for instance, penetrates more or less in a straight line toward the dentinoenamel junction.

At the bottom of occlusal fissures or pits the picture is different. Here the enamel rods still lie nearly perpendicular to the dentinoenamel junction, but the sharp concavity of the junction in these locations results in a radial pattern—a fanning out—of the rods (Fig. 18). The caries lesion starting in the fissure or pit and penetrating in the direction of the rod length, radiates

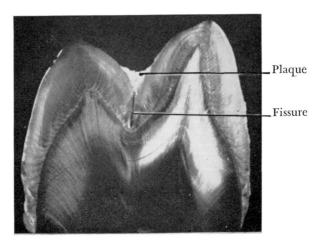

Figure 31. Ground section through a maxillary first premolar tooth cut buccolingually. The central developmental groove has a deep fissure at its base. The thin enamel at the bottom of the fissure seems to be intact, but the appearance of the dentin immediately beneath it suggests that caries was present in the fissure at one side or the other of the section here seen, and that the lesion had spread near the dentinoenamel junction, undermining the sound surface enamel. A dense plaque is present in the groove, but in this particular area it seems not to be dense enough within the fissure to be visible in the photomicrograph.

as it deepens (Fig. 32). The result is a deceptive clinical picture. Clinical examination may reveal only a small carious area visible in a developmental groove; but at the dentinoenamel junction, invisible without x-ray pictures, the broadening of the lesion has left the surface enamel unsupported (Figs. 33, 34A and B).

While fissures and pits are commonly thought of as occurring on occlusal surfaces of molar and premolar teeth, they are found also in other places. In some molar teeth pits are found at the cervical end of buccal developmental grooves (Figs. 17 and 111). Examine Figure 35A and B. The pit at the end of the buccal groove (Fig. 35A) has a caries lesion, not obvious from the outside, that penetrates some distance into the dentin (Fig. 35B).

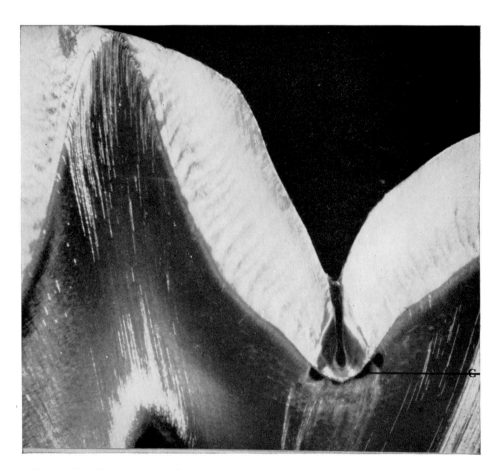

Figure 32. Ground section of a molar tooth. The fissure in the occlusal developmental groove clearly is affected by dental caries. Notice the radiating pattern of the lesion in the enamel near the bottom of the fissure. This is due to the fanning out of the enamel rods. (See Figure 18.) The dentin beneath the bottom of the fissure is destroyed near the dentinoenamel junction (C), leaving the enamel unsupported. There is little evidence of sclerosis of the dentin beneath this lesion. The bacteria here have probably penetrated well into the dentinal tubules (Chapter 4). The plaque is indistinctly seen in this ground section. Often plaques are destroyed in the process of grinding the section. Notice attrition on the cusp tip.

Figure 33. Ground section of a molar tooth. In this tooth the caries started in the enamel at the bottom of the fissure and spread along the dentinoenamel junction. In this area the lesion has visibly penetrated the dentin, and the effect of caries is seen in the dentin over a broad area at the dentinoenamel junction and pulpward. The dark region in the dentin beneath the fissure, broad near the dentinoenamel junction and more narrow nearer the pulp, is carious dentin (see Chapter 4). Caries will spread downward, destroying the unaffected dentin beneath it and around it. Destruction of dentin will leave the superficial enamel unsupported.

Figure 34. A. Even the casual observer can see that this mandibular first molar is carious in the occlusal fissures. The extent of the lesion is partly seen when the distolingual portion of the tooth (asterisk) is ground off. B. Caries has probably penetrated farther into the dentin in an area beyond the cut surface here seen. Under the triangular ridge of the distal cusp caries in the dentin has noticeably undermined the enamel.

Figure 35. A. Clearly there is caries in the occlusal grooves of this mandibular second molar. The buccal pit at the end of the buccal groove appears to be deep but undamaged. Removal of the mesial side of the tooth (asterisk) reveals considerable caries damage B in the buccal pit and a deep penetration into the occlusal dentin beneath the bucco-occlusal groove.

Figure 36. A maxillary first molar with a prominent cusp of Carabelli was ground to reveal the deep fissure at the line of attachment of this fifth cusp to the mesiolingual cusp. In this tooth the enamel of the fissure appears to be intact. In some similar fissures, caries is present. (The cusp of Carabelli is at the left of the picture. The oblong object at the right is part of an amalgam filling in the occlusal surface.)

Again, at the junction of the cusp of Carabelli and the mesiolingual cusp of the maxillary molar to which it is attached there is a groove, often deep enough to be called a fissure, which is susceptible to caries (Fig. 36).

Unexpectedly, a pit may be present at the incisal border of the cingulum of a maxillary incisor tooth that has a deep lingual fossa and heavy marginal ridges. This was the external appearance of the maxillary central incisor pictured in Figure 37. A ground section of this tooth reveals a deep developmental depression. Such an invagination is at times so deep that it protrudes into the pulp cavity. It is called a *dens in dente* (a tooth in a tooth). Notice that enamel lines the surface of this invagination.

In some mongoloid peoples deep grooves, oriented apicoincisally, occur characteristically on the cingulum of mandibular incisors. In such places caries often develops.

Surprisingly, pits often are on the incisal edges of mandibular incisor teeth when there are prominent mamelons. The pits seen in Figure 38 are not

Figure 37. This maxillary central incisor had a deep lingual fossa, pronounced marginal ridges, and what appeared to be a pit at the incisal border of the cingulum. It was ground to a thin center section. In this photomicrograph what appeared to be a small lingual pit is seen to extend deep into the tooth and to be lined with a thin layer of enamel. No caries was evident in this tooth even when the section was examined under high magnification. However, caries frequently is found in such invaginations. In some teeth this kind of developmental invagination is much deeper, and is called *dens in dente* (tooth within a tooth).

Figure 38. Ground section of a mandibular incisor tooth cut mesiodistally. The intact tooth had mamelons that appeared unusually pronounced. The ground section shows deep pits in the depressions between the mamelons, with a very thin layer of enamel at the bottom of the pits. In making ground sections of a number of teeth that had unusually pronounced mamelons, it was found that such pits were generally present. Notice the curvature of the dentinal tubules in the tooth crown. In the root the tubules are nearly straight and are directed slightly apically from the cementodentinal junction.

carious, but sometimes in such pits early caries can be detected in the study of a ground section.

With these several structural characteristics of enamel tending to facilitate the spread of caries beneath the enamel surface, it is easy to see how one day an individual may bite on something firm and part of the surface of a seemingly (to the patient) good tooth will cave in. An understanding of the subsurface spread of dental caries* motivates the dentist and the dental hygienist to instruct patients of the importance of regular dental examinations and of the necessity for prompt attention to even seemingly small cavities.

* A word about the term *dental caries: Caries* is the correct form of the word. You may say that a person has caries; or that he has a carious tooth; or that he has a cavity in a tooth. Or you may say that caries *is* (singular verb) present in a mouth. But you never say a person has "a carie"—any more than you say a person has a *measle* or a *mump*.

CHAPTER 4

Dentin

Dentin is located in both the crown and the root of a tooth, making up the bulk of the tooth. In an intact tooth the dentin is not visible because in the crown it is covered by enamel and in the root it is covered by cementum (Figs. 15 and 39).

COMPOSITION

Dentin is a calcified tissue, and like all calcified tissues of the body it is composed of both *organic* and *inorganic* (mineral) substances. Although not nearly so hard as tooth enamel, dentin is harder than bone. Mature dentin is about 70 per cent inorganic substance and about 30 per cent organic material and water. (Compare these figures with those given for enamel in Chapter 3.)

STRUCTURE OF DENTIN

The organic matrix of dentin is composed of very small fibrils and their surrounding structureless cementing substance. During the development of dentin the organic matrix is formed first, and then minerals in solution are deposited in its cementing substance. The minerals crystallize out of solution, the crystals forming on and around the minute fibrils. Thus dentin becomes a hard tissue. The mineral substance of dentin is similar to the mineral substance of enamel, cementum, and bone.

Dentin is perforated by innumerable holes called *dentinal tubules* which contain *dentinal fibers* (not to be confused with the *fibrils* of the dentin matrix). The dentinal tubules lie close together and extend from the tooth pulp to the dentinoenamel junction in the crown of the tooth and to the dentinocemental junction in the root (Figs. 1, 12 and 21). At their outer ends the dentinal tubules are divided into a number of branches (Figs. 26 and 27). Much smaller branches connecting adjacent dentinal tubules are often found along the length of the tubules. In diameter (Fig. 40) the dentinal tubules measure about 3 microns at the pulpal ends and somewhat less at the outer ends. In the cusp tips in the tooth crown (Fig. 33) and in the apical half of the root (Figs. 38 and 39) the dentinal tubules are nearly straight and are arranged nearly perpendicular to the dentinoenamel or dentinocemental junction. In the facial, lingual, mesial, and distal areas of the crown (Figs. 29 and 38) and in the cervical portion of the roots (Fig. 39) the dentinal tubules are S-shaped. The outer ends of the S-shaped tubules are always occlusal to the pulpal ends of the tubules.

Figure 39. A photomicrograph of a ground section cut faciolingually through a maxillary first molar tooth. This tooth is shown diagrammatically in Figure 15.

Figure 40. A photomicrograph of a ground section of dentin cut in such a direction that the dentinal tubules are seen in cross section. The specimen was dipped in a histologic stain which remained in the tubules, making them appear dark in the picture. The tubules in this section, taken from near the pulp of the tooth (rather than close to the enamel), are probably about 3 microns in diameter.

A *dentinal fiber* (also called a *Tomes'* fiber*) occupies each dentinal tubule (Figs. 25 and 41). A dentinal fiber is the cytoplasm of a pulp cell. Those cells of the pulp which lie next to the dentin have the somewhat surprising distinction of being cells of the dentin also. They are named *odontoblasts*. The nucleus of the odontoblast cell remains in the pulp surrounded by part of the cell's cytoplasm. The remainder of the cytoplasm of the odontoblast cell is stretched out like a long, thin tail and extends into a dentinal tubule (Figs. 41 and 53). This cytoplasmic extension of the odontoblast is called a dentinal fiber (Tomes' fiber). Each dentinal fiber extends through the tubule to the dentinoenamel or dentinocemental junction. At their peripheral ends near the dentinoenamel and dentinocemental junctions the dentinal fibers are branched just as the dentinal tubules are branched (Fig. 41).

In some places in the crown of a tooth the peripheral ends of some dentinal fibers cross the dentinoenamel junction and protrude into the enamel. Here they appear as short, slightly thickened structures. These ends of dentinal fibers in the enamel are *enamel spindles* (Figs. 25, 26, 27 and 41).

In the crowns of some teeth the dentin has in it spots which are uncalcified or are hypocalcified (hypo = under, less than ordinary). These uncalcified spots, irregular in shape, usually occur in a layer a short distance inside the dentinoenamel junction (Figs. 12, 13, 14, 42 and 56). In this location such areas of uncalcified dentin are called *interglobular dentin*. The reason for the

* Pronounced *Tōmz*.

Figure 41. A diagrammatic illustration of a small portion of tooth pulp showing the structure of the pulp and the relation of the odontoblast cells of the pulp to the dentin and the enamel. **A.** Tooth pulp as seen under high power magnification. **B.** Diagrammatic illustration of the small enclosed area shown in A. The odontoblast cells of the pulp have cytoplasmic processes, the dentinal fibers, which extend in the dentinal tubules to the dentinoenamel junction. The fibers are branched at their peripheral ends. The portion of the odontoblast process that crosses the dentinoenamel junction into the enamel is an enamel spindle.

failure of proper calcification here is probably some metabolic disturbance which occurred at the time this part of the tooth was forming.

Root dentin invariably contains a band of minute uncalcified spots almost immediately beneath the cementum. This is called *Tomes' granular layer* (Figs. 12, 13, 14, 15, 43, 56 and 59). It was first described by the dental histologist Sir John Tomes (1815–1895) who thought that this region of the dentin had a granular appearance. Later it was found that this area is not really granular, but is made up of very small uncalcified spots in the dentin. Tomes' granular layer has considerable clinical importance which will be discussed later.

In the root dentin of some teeth a short distance beneath Tomes' granular layer there may be also a layer of interglobular dentin similar in size and configuration to the interglobular dentin found in the crown of the tooth (Fig. 43).

Enamel

Dentinoenamel
junction

Dentin

Interglobular
dentin

Figure 42. Photomicrograph of part of a ground section of a tooth crown. The enamel is divided from the dentin at the scalloped dentinoenamel junction. Curvatures in the enamel rods are evident and in some areas cross-striations of the rods can be seen. In the dentin at the bottom of the picture are irregular areas (dark) of interglobular dentin.

A modified type of dentin known as *secondary dentin* is usually found in older teeth along the pulpal wall of the dentin. Aside from the fact that in varying degrees it has fewer and less regular dentinal tubules than the first dentin produced, secondary dentin is similar to the earlier dentin. Secondary dentin may be formed throughout the life of the tooth as long as the pulp is intact.

In certain areas on the pulpal wall secondary dentin is formed in larger amounts. In posterior teeth it is formed in larger amounts in the pulp horn—that is, in the part of the pulp that extends toward the cusp tips—and on the floor of the pulp chamber (Figs. 14, 15, 45, 54). In anterior teeth it is formed in larger amounts beneath the incisal edge when there has been considerable attrition (wearing off) (Fig. 44). It may occur in larger amounts also on the pulpal wall in areas where dental caries has penetrated to the dentinoenamel junction (Figs. 15 and 55). Its greater formation in these areas is often a result of the reaction of the tooth pulp to the irritation of attrition or caries.

Because secondary dentin produced in response to attrition, caries, operative procedures, or other damaging stimuli usually has fewer and more irregular dentinal tubules than secondary dentin ordinarily produced merely as a result of aging, this dentin is often referred to as *irregular dentin* instead of as secondary dentin.

Sclerotic dentin is a modified dentin found in some areas of most old teeth and sometimes in young teeth. Dentin is said to be sclerotic when the dentinal fibers have degenerated and the dentinal tubules have become filled with cal-

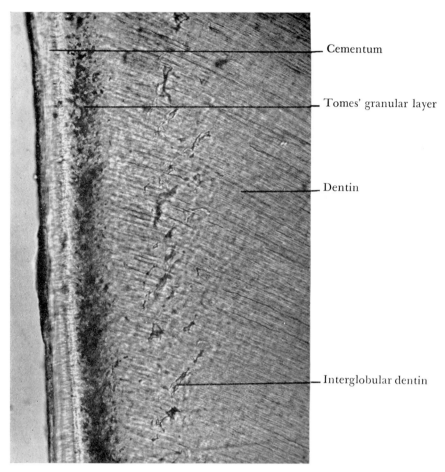

Cementum

Tomes' granular layer

Dentin

Interglobular dentin

Figure 43. Photomicrograph of part of a ground section of tooth root. The cementum is the relatively narrow light band at the left of the picture; the dentin is the wide area at the right of the picture. In the dentin close to the cementum is the band of closely packed small areas of uncalcified dentin called Tomes' granular layer. Deeper in the dentin are larger, irregular areas of interglobular dentin (dark areas). Notice that the dentinal tubules are straight, and are not quite at right angles to the cementodentinal junction. In the cementum are small lines, perpendicular to the cementum surface, which are spaces once occupied by Sharpey's fibers (Chapter 6). (High power magnification.)

Figure 44. Photomicrograph of a ground section (cut faciolingually) of a canine tooth. Extensive attrition has resulted in the loss of the enamel and part of the dentin of the cusp. The formation of secondary dentin in the incisal part of the pulp cavity has protected the pulp from exposure.

Figure 45. Photomicrograph of a ground section of a mandibular molar tooth. A large amount of secondary dentin has formed in the pulp horns of both the buccal and lingual cusps. Notice the attrition of the enamel on the cusp tips.

cium salts. Sclerotic dentin is often found beneath worn enamel such as occurs in the incisal area of anterior teeth, and beneath slowly progressing dental caries in locations where secondary dentin is being produced on the pulpal wall (Fig. 15). Sclerotic dentin is also found beneath Tomes' granular layer in the cervical area of older teeth where the cervical cementum has become exposed to the oral cavity as a result of recession of the gingiva (Chapter 10).

In the mandibular incisor tooth shown in Figure 46 the dentinal fibers have degenerated beneath the worn incisal edge, but the dentinal tubules have not become filled with calcium salts. Such an area has been referred to as a *dead tract*. The pulp beneath the dead tract in this tooth is protected by the presence of secondary dentin.

At the cervix on the facial side of this tooth there is a change in the dentin beneath the cervical abrasion. The white area, indicated by the pointer, is probably a dead tract. Outside of the dead tract, nearer the surface of the tooth, the dentin appears to be sclerotic—*i.e.*, the tubules are filled, or are becoming filled, with calcium salts.

CLINICAL IMPORTANCE OF THE STRUCTURE OF DENTIN

The structure of dentin influences both the pattern of a caries lesion and the speed with which dental caries destroys a tooth; and it accounts for the sensitivity frequently experienced by patients during the performance of an oral prophylaxis or during the eating of hot or cold foods.

In the preceding chapter it was explained that dental caries is a disease of the hard tissues of the tooth: acidogenic bacteria convert sugars into acids which dissolve the minerals out of the hard tooth tissues; and proteolytic (protein-destroying) bacteria destroy the organic component of the hard tooth tissue in the same area.

When at any point the caries process has penetrated the enamel to the depth of the dentinoenamel junction, the caries-producing bacteria will also reach this depth and will come in contact with the peripheral ends of the dentinal tubules. Since the bacteria are smaller than the diameter of the dentinal tubules they enter the tubules. The dentinal fibers which occupy the tubules are destroyed. The bacteria travel pulpward in the opened tubules and the dentin is slowly destroyed. Because the bacteria follow the course of the dentinal tubules, a caries lesion originating around a contact area or in the cervical area of a tooth extends in an apical direction as it approaches the pulp. Notice the direction of the dentinal tubules in Figures 15, 39, and 46.

The horizontal spread of caries is considerably more rapid in dentin than in enamel. A tooth with only a small area of caries visible on its surface may be so extensively carious in the dentin that clinical restoration is impossible. It is not difficult to understand why the teeth shown in Figures 47*A* and *B*, and 48*A* and *B* were lost. The occlusal surface of these teeth, particularly 47*A*, showed too little damage to impress even an observing patient with the probably serious condition inside the tooth.

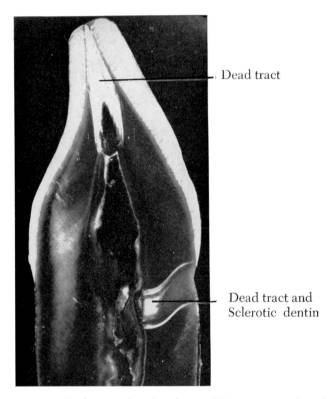

Dead tract

Dead tract and
Sclerotic dentin

Figure 46.   Photomicrograph of a ground section of a mandibular incisor tooth cut faciolingually Beneath the worn incisal edge is a dead tract in the dentin.   Deposition of secondary dentin beneath the dead tract has protected the pulp from damage.   On the facial side of the tooth in the cervical area there is abrasion: the cementum is gone and some of the dentin has been worn away. (See Chapter 10, Figure 97.)   Beneath this abraded surface there is an alteration in the dentin.   Near the pulp is an area of dead tract, which appears white.   Superficial (nearer the surface) to this tract the dentin seems to be sclerotic.   On the pulp wall in this region secondary dentin has been produced; it protrudes into the pulp cavity inside the dead tract.   Notice the curvature of the dentinal tubules in the cervical area.

Figure 47. A. This maxillary molar shows evidence of caries in the central fossa and in the mesial triangular fossa, but the casual observer scarcely expects what is revealed when the buccal side of the tooth (asterisk) is ground away. B. Caries has penetrated to the pulp cavity and has spread laterally, undermining the enamel of the entire occlusal surface. (Notice the curvatures of the dentinal tubules.)

Figure 48. A. This maxillary molar was clearly carious in the central fossa, and probably also in the groove between the lingual cusps. Removal of the distobuccal side of the tooth (asterisk) exposed a deep lesion in the central fossa (B), but little evidence of caries in the distolingual groove at this particular point. The groove may have been carious either buccal to or lingual to the area we see here.

The teeth shown in Figures 49*A* and *B*, 50*A* and *B*, and 51*A* and *B* had a larger surface area of visible caries, and the enamel around the point of entry was so seriously undermined that a large part of it was unsupported. With this kind of condition, the occlusal enamel often collapses completely when the patient bites on some relatively soft food.

Figure 49. A. Caries is obvious in the central fossa of this maxillary molar, and an area of possible caries is seen in the lingual developmental groove. When the mesial surface of the tooth was removed (asterisk) completely unsupported enamel was exposed around the central fossa and around the suspicious area in the groove B. Notice the extent of caries in the dentin.

The progress of dental caries through the dentin is often retarded, but not stopped, by defense reactions that take place in the pulp. One such reaction is the production of *sclerotic dentin*. From the pulp tissue calcium salts are deposited in the dentinal tubules causing them to become filled with mineral substances, and so the progress of bacterial invasion is slowed down. Another defense reaction against caries is the formation by the pulp of additional dentin, called *secondary dentin*, at the location where the bacteria-filled tubules reach the pulp. This increases the thickness of the dentin wall and helps to

Figure 50. A. The extent of destruction beneath the occlusal surface of this maxillary molar is seen when the distal side of the tooth (asterisk) has been removed B. The occlusal enamel is undermined around the occlusal opening of the lesion. Caries has penetrated also from the lingual developmental groove.

protect the tooth pulp, for a time at least, against the invasion of the disease. In a tooth from which the pulp has been removed these defense changes which are dependent upon the pulp cannot occur.

Another characteristic of dentin of particular interest to dentist and dental hygienist is the location of Tomes' granular layer and its effect on the comfort of the patient. As we have seen, Tomes' granular layer consists of a narrow band of uncalcified areas in the root dentin immediately beneath the cementum. A natural aging process which occurs in nearly all mouths is the gradual recession of the gingiva and a resulting exposure of the cementum at the necks of the teeth. (This will be discussed in Chapter 10.) In the performance of an oral prophylaxis it is necessary to clean this exposed cervical cementum. This means working very close to Tomes' granular layer which, being uncalcified and in close contact with the dentinal fibers, causes this area to be very sensitive. Therefore the patient may experience pain. The patient may also find this area of exposed cementum sensitive to hot or cold foods. A patient with exposed cervical cementum may believe that he has caries in this area because of the pain he experiences during eating or while brushing his teeth. These discomforts are more noticeable when the cervical cementum first becomes exposed. After the cervical cementum has been exposed to the oral environment for a few weeks or months the dentin beneath the exposed surface usually becomes sclerotic (Fig. 46) and the patient ceases to notice discomfort.

Figure 51. A. This mandibular second molar has caries in the central fossa. Removal of the lingual side of the tooth (asterisk) exposed a lesion in the dentin that extended horizontally beneath enamel that on the surface appeared undamaged B.

CHAPTER 5

Tooth Pulp

LOCATION

The pulp of a tooth is located in the interior of the tooth. It occupies the pulp chamber in the crown and the root canal in the root of the tooth, and connects with the periodontal ligament at the apical foramen (Fig. 13).

COMPOSITION

Tooth pulp is the only noncalcified tissue of a tooth. It is a soft connective tissue, and like other connective tissues it is made up of *cells* and *intercellular substance* (Fig. 52). In young teeth the cells of the pulp tissue are more numerous than they are in older teeth and the intercellular substance is relatively smaller in amount.

While the *cells* of young pulp tissue are chiefly *fibroblasts*, specialized types of cells also are present: *histiocytes, undifferentiated mesenchymal cells, odontoblasts.*

The *intercellular substance* of the pulp consists of two kinds of material, the *amorphous substance* (a = not; morphous = form; *i.e.* structureless) and the *fibrous substance*. The amorphous substance is a jelly-like material in which are suspended all of the cellular and fibrous elements of the pulp tissue. The fibrous substance is a meshwork of minute fibrils. In the peripheral part of young pulp the fibrous substance is massed into little coiled, rope-like bundles called *Korff's fibers.*

Tooth pulp contains *blood vessels* and *nerves*. In many teeth there are also calcified structures called *denticles* (pulp stones) and *diffuse calcifications.*

STRUCTURES IN THE PULP

Fibroblast cells are more numerous than any other kind of cell in the pulp (Fig. 52). Often they are described as star-shaped because of the irregular pointed outlines of their cytoplasm. Fibroblasts are responsible for the formation of the intercellular substance of pulp tissue.

Histiocytes and *undifferentiated mesenchymal cells* are located throughout the pulp near the capillaries. They are part of the pulp's defense mechanism and they respond to pulp injury by changing into defense cells of the sorts seen in any inflammatory reaction.

The *odontoblasts* are specialized fibroblasts which are located next to the dentin (Fig. 52). They are roughly cylindrical in shape, being somewhat longer than they are wide, and they contain an oval-shaped nucleus. They are peculiar cells in that their cytoplasm does not remain entirely in the pulp. While part of the cytoplasm of the odontoblast remains surrounding the

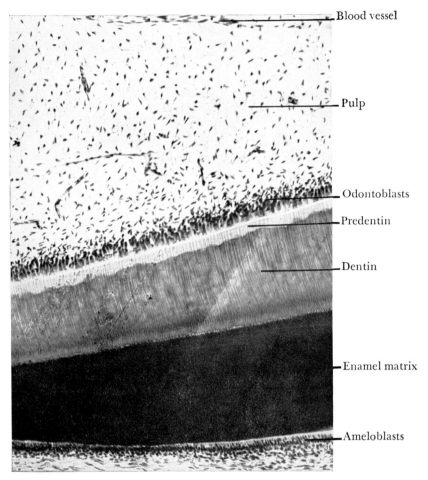

Blood vessel

Pulp

Odontoblasts

Predentin

Dentin

Enamel matrix

Ameloblasts

Figure 52. A section through a developing tooth of a pig. The tissues are very similar to those of a human tooth. The dark-stained, as yet uncalcified, enamel matrix is covered on its outer surface by the layer of ameloblasts which are beginning to lose their columnar shape. (See Chapter 11.) The dentin contains dentinal tubules which extend from the dentinoenamel junction to the pulp. The layer of dentin next to the pulp is uncalcified, and is called predentin, or dentinoid. In this section it is stained a lighter color than the earlier formed, calcified dentin. The pulp cells next to the predentin are the odontoblasts. Most of the other cells seen in the pulp are fibroblasts. Korff's fibers are not seen in this preparation. They require a special stain. Nerves are not seen in this preparation. Small blood vessels are scattered throughout the pulp tissue, and a larger blood vessel is seen at the top of the picture.

nucleus in the usual manner of cells, the remainder of it is stretched out in a long, thin tail which enters a dentinal tubule and extends in the tubule to the dentinoenamel or the dentinocemental junction (Figs. 41 and 53). This cytoplasmic tail of the odontoblast is called a *dentinal fiber* (*Tomes' fiber*). When a dentinal fiber crosses the dentinoenamel junction into the enamel, the portion of it that is in the enamel is called an *enamel spindle* (Figs. 25, 26, 27, and 41).

Korff's fibers are minute rope-like, corkscrew-shaped structures which lie among the odontoblasts. They are produced by the merging of the fibrils of the fibrous intercellular substance of the pulp. Korff's fibers may be made visible for microscopic examination by special staining techniques applied to thin sections of young pulp tissue. They seem to have an important function in the formation of the dentin matrix. (See Chapter 11.)

Blood vessels are plentiful in young pulp (Fig. 52). Small branches from the superior or the inferior alveolar artery enter the tooth through the apical foramen. They pass through the root canal to the pulp chamber and divide into capillaries. The circulating blood is collected into veins which pass out from the pulp through the apical foramen. *Lymphatic vessels* also have been demonstrated in the pulp.

Along with the blood vessels, *nerves* enter the tooth through the apical foramen, giving the pulp a rich nerve supply. The maxillary teeth are supplied by branches from the second division, and the mandibular teeth by branches from the third division of the trigeminal nerve. At the inner ends of the odontoblast cells the nerves in the pulp form a network, with some

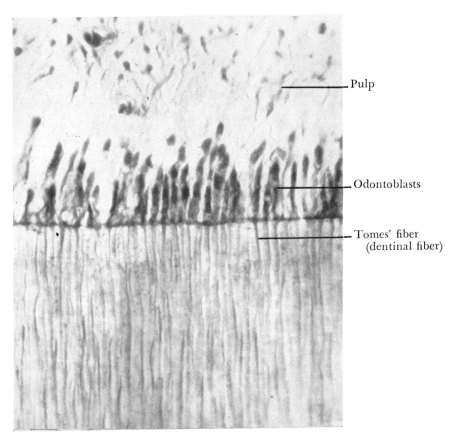

Figure 53. A section through the pulp and predentin of a young human tooth. The odontoblasts are dark-stained columnar cells. The nuclei and part of the cytoplasm of the odontoblasts are in the pulp. Long fibers of cytoplasm extend into the dentinal tubules. These are the *dentinal fibers,* or *Tomes' fibers.*

nerve fibers having endings on the odontoblasts. This arrangement helps to account for the sensitivity of the dentin, since the odontoblasts have part of their cytoplasm in the dentinal tubules. Some investigators have demonstrated structures in the dentinal tubules which they have identified as nerves.

Denticles are calcified structures of an irregularly rounded shape commonly found in tooth pulp (Figs. 15 and 54). They may lie free in the soft tissue or they may be attached to the dentin wall. They vary in shape and size, the size increasing with the age of the tooth. Generally they are regarded as of little clinical importance excepting as they may interfere with endodontic treatment. They are never a source of infection.

Diffuse calcifications are small, thin scatterings of calcified material frequently found in the pulps of older teeth, usually in the root canals (Figs. 15 and 55). Clinically they are usually unimportant.

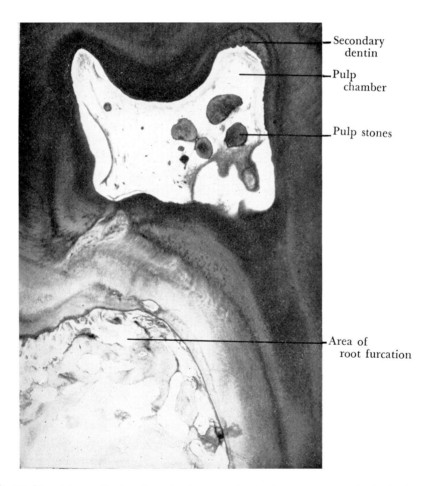

Figure 54. A longitudinal section of a human molar tooth. This was an old tooth. The soft pulp tissue has been shrunken and damaged in the preparation of the tissue, but the denticles (pulp stones) are clearly seen. Secondary dentin is seen in the pulp horns. This section was cut at such an angle that it does not pass through the narrow root canal, but of course a root canal was present. The lower left corner of the picture is the area of the root furcation.

FUNCTIONS OF THE PULP

Tooth pulp has several functions. For purposes of description these functions may be listed as follows: (1) formative, (2) sensory, (3) nutritive, (4)
defensive.

The *formative function*. Tooth pulp produces the dentin of the tooth, as
will be explained in the discussion of tooth development to be found in
Chapter 11. We will see that Korff's fibers, which are composed of the fibrillar
material of the intercellular substance, give rise to the fibrils of the dentin
matrix. The pulp also produces the amorphous cementing substance of the
dentin matrix. And the odontoblast cells of the pulp have their cytoplasm
stretched out into thin, thread-like extensions which are the dentinal fibers
that occupy the dentinal tubules.

The *sensory function*. Tooth pulp is sensitive to external stimuli. The nerves
in the pulp are responsible for some of the sensation experienced by an individual when a stimulus is applied to the tooth. It is an interesting fact that
the sensation educed by stimuli received by a tooth pulp is a sensation of
pain. A person cannot differentiate between extremes of heat (hot coffee)
and of cold (ice cream) applied to the tooth. If sensation is experienced it is
merely pain in either case. Slight pressures on a tooth will produce a sensation of pressure or touch. Most of this sensation is due to pressure on the
periodontal ligament.

The *nutritive function*. Since tooth pulp is a living tissue with a blood supply,
it receives nutrients from the blood stream. It may be supposed that nutrients
enter the dentinal tubules either by way of the cytoplasmic dentinal fibers or
around the outside of the dentinal fibers. Such nutrients may be carried in
this way as far as the dentinoenamel and dentinocemental junctions. There
is a good deal yet to be learned about this subject.

Since unwarranted deductions are sometimes made from a set of briefly
presented facts such as those given above, it should be made clear that whatever the manner of nutrition of the dentin this is a matter entirely apart from
the question of dental caries. We cannot associate the nutritive function of
the pulp and the general nutrition of the individual with the presence or
absence of dental caries activity. Such association should not be attempted
from the above discussion. Dental caries is a disease which starts on the outside surface of the tooth and is a process of an entirely different nature.

The *defensive function*. Defense reactions of the pulp are expressed in several
ways: pulp may show an inflammatory reaction; pulp may change the character of existing dentin (sclerosis); pulp may produce additional dentin
(secondary dentin).

In case of pulp damage the pulp shows an inflammatory reaction. Cells
appear which are commonly found at any site of inflammation. Some of
these defense cells are derived from histiocytes and undifferentiated mesenchymal cells of the pulp; some are carried into the pulp by the blood stream from
their points of origin in the bone marrow and lymph nodes. As the defense
cells become effective in controlling the damaging process, the pulp may
produce sclerosis of the existing dentin and may also lay down secondary
dentin along the pulpal wall.

Sclerosis (sclero = hard) of the dentin involves the filling in of the dentinal tubules, usually in a restricted area, with calcium salts so that the dentin in this area is a solid calcified tissue instead of a tissue perforated with tubules which contain dentinal fibers (Fig. 15). Sclerotic dentin usually occurs beneath a caries lesion and its presence tends to retard the progress of the destruction of the tooth tissue. The stimulus to the pulp which causes the dentine sclerosis is received through the dentinal tubules.

Pulpal to the sclerotic dentin the pulp may produce, as a defense reaction, varying amounts of *secondary dentin* which gives the pulp additional protection against external irritation. The formation of secondary dentin and sclerotic dentin occur in aging teeth, where infection is not a factor, as a result of the stimulation produced by attrition (Fig 46).

Age Changes in the Pulp

Just as age brings about changes in other parts of the body, it brings about changes in the pulps of teeth. These changes are universal and normal and are not to be regarded as pathologic. The continued formation of secondary dentin with increasing age causes the pulp chamber to become smaller and the root canals to become narrower. In some old teeth which show heavy attrition or dental caries of long standing, the pulp chamber may be entirely filled by the deposition of secondary dentin. The cells of the pulp, very numerous in young teeth, decrease in number with age, and the fibrous intercellular substance is relatively increased. Old tooth pulps are composed mostly of fibrous intercellular substance. The blood supply of the pulp decreases with age. Denticles are larger and more numerous in old teeth and diffuse calcifications are increased. These changes of the pulp do not alter the function of the tooth.

Clinical Importance of the Pulp

A fully developed tooth may function for many years after its pulp has been removed and the pulp canal filled. Although the enamel of the tooth becomes more brittle, its function is not affected by the loss of the pulp. The cementum is not affected, nor is the process of continued cementum formation. A tooth without a pulp cannot, however, produce secondary dentin or sclerotic dentin. Loss of a tooth pulp usually comes about as a result of caries or of tooth fracture, with accompanying pulp infection. Careful treatment by the dentist is essential in either case to prevent the infection from traveling through the root canal and apical foramen into the tissues surrounding the tooth, with possibly a consequent loss of the tooth.

CHAPTER 6

Cementum

LOCATION

Cementum is the layer of calcified tissue, about .05 mm. thick at the tooth cervix, which makes up the surface of the root of a tooth (Figs. 12, 43, and 56). It overlies and is attached to the root dentin. In the area of the cemento-enamel junction the cementum may have any one of three relationships with the enamel of the tooth crown: it may exactly meet the enamel; it may not quite meet the enamel, leaving a little dentin exposed; or it may slightly over-lap the enamel (Figs. 12, 14, 55, 56, 57, and 58). This last arrangement is the most common.

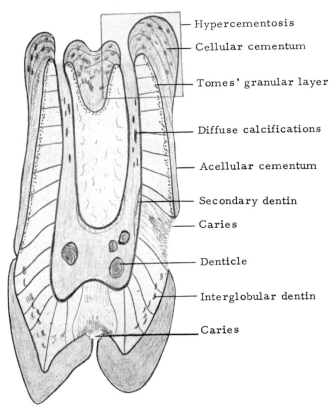

— Hypercementosis

— Cellular cementum

— Tomes' granular layer

— Diffuse calcifications

— Acellular cementum

— Secondary dentin

— Caries

— Denticle

— Interglobular dentin

— Caries

Figure 55. Diagrammatic drawing of a longitudinal faciolingual section of a maxillary first premolar tooth. The tip of the lingual root shows a very large amount of cementum, which is some-times referred to as hypercementosis. For a photomicrograph of such thick cementum see Figures 59 and 61.

COMPOSITION

Like enamel, dentin, and bone, cementum is made up of *organic matrix* which contains crystallized mineral substances. Cementum may have cells, called *cementocytes*, irregularly scattered through it. It does not contain blood vessels or nerves. Cementum is not quite so hard as dentin, being about 50 per cent inorganic (mineral) material and about 50 per cent organic substance and water. This is about the same hardness as bone.

STRUCTURE OF CEMENTUM

Compared to the structure of dentin, cementum has some similarities and some differences. As in dentin, the organic matrix is composed of a frame-

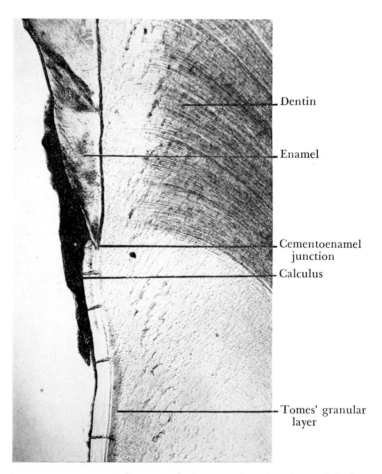

Figure 56. A photomicrograph (low power) of a ground section of a tooth in the area of the cementoenamel junction. The cementum overlaps the enamel slightly. Calculus adheres to both the enamel and the cementum. The four conspicuous lines in the cementum are cracks produced by the grinding of the section. Tomes' granular layer lies beneath the cementum in the dentin. Deeper in the dentin in both the root and the crown are irregular dark areas of interglobular dentin. The dentinal tubules are distinct. The darkness of the tubules in the upper right is a result of air in the tubules due to the preparation of the section; it is not due to any structural change.

work of fine fibrils held together by an amorphous cementing substance which becomes calcified. Unlike dentin, cementum may contain whole cells. You will recall that dentin contains processes of pulp cells but it does not contain entire cells.

Cementum is a product of the periodontal ligament, which is the layer of connective tissue that lies between the tooth root and the bony socket in which the root is set (Fig. 66). Certain cells of the periodontal ligament (*cemento-blasts*) lying close to the tooth root become converted into cells of the cementum (*cementocytes*) as the cementum is being formed.

Cementocytes are connected with one another by numerous thread-like projections of their cytoplasm. The space in the cementum which is occupied by the body of the cementocyte is called a *lacuna* (little space); and the spaces occupied by the cytoplasmic projections of the cementocyte are called *canaliculi* (little canals). Canaliculi of adjacent lacunae may join and thus

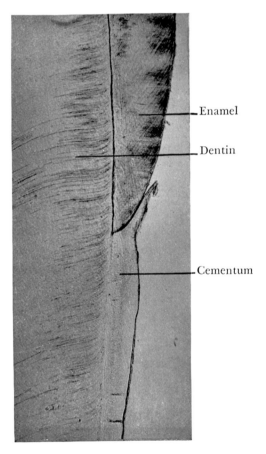

Enamel

Dentin

Cementum

Figure 57. A photomicrograph of a ground section of a tooth in the area of the cemento-enamel junction. The cementum overlaps the enamel considerably. The separation of the cementum from the enamel at the border of the cementum is an artifact probably caused by the drying of the specimen during preparation of the section; in life the cementum was no doubt fixed firmly against the enamel surface;

connect neighboring lacunae. In cementum most of the canaliculi are directed toward the periodontal ligament (Figs. 12, 13, 59, and 60).

Ordinarily cementocytes are not found throughout the entire cementum on the tooth root. Usually the thin cementum on the cervical portion of the root has no cementocytes. In the apical portion of the root the cementum is usually relatively thick, and while in this region the cementum close to the dentin may have few cementocytes, the outer layers often contain many irregularly distributed cementocytes. Cementum which contains cementocytes is called *cellular cementum*, and cementum which has no cementocytes is called *acellular cementum* (Figs. 12, 13, 14, 55, 59, and 60).

The outer surface of cementum, next to the periodontal ligament, remains less calcified than the rest of the cementum and is called *cementoid*.

Visible in the cementum by microscopic examination are structures called

Figure 58. A photomicrograph of a ground section of a tooth in the area of the cemento-enamel junction. The cementum on this tooth overlaps the enamel to an unusual extent. Not many teeth show this amount of overlapping. The separation of the cementum from the enamel is probably due to the drying of the specimen during preparation. In life the cementum undoubtedly was firm against the enamel. This is the mesial side of a mandibular molar tooth.

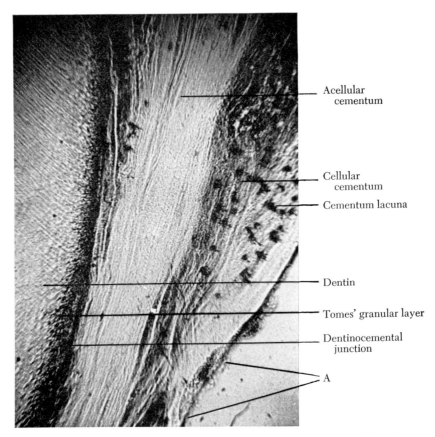

Acellular cementum

Cellular cementum

Cementum lacuna

Dentin

Tomes' granular layer

Dentinocemental junction

A

Figure 59. A photomicrograph of an area of thick cementum on a tooth root. Taken from an area similar to that shown at the tip of the lingual root of the tooth in Figure 55. A indicates the surface of the tooth root to which the periodontal ligament was attached.

Sharpey's fibers (Figs. 43 and 63). These are the ends of bundles of fibers of the periodontal ligament which have become embedded in the cementum during its formation. They attach the periodontal ligament firmly to the tooth.

CLINICAL IMPORTANCE OF CEMENTUM

The cementum is part of the mechanism by which a tooth is attached in the tooth socket. Just as the periodontal ligament is attached to the tooth by Sharpey's fibers embedded in the cementum, it is similarly attached to the tooth socket by Sharpey's fibers embedded in the bone (Figs. 62, 63, and 64). The result of this double attachment is that the tooth is literally suspended in its socket (Chapter 7).

Cementum probably continues to be produced intermittently by the periodontal ligament throughout the life of the tooth. Additions of cementum at the root apex are believed to cause a slow occlusal movement of the tooth that partially compensates for the loss of crown length which results from attrition during years of use.

Cementum also repairs damage to the tooth root: it may replace lost areas

Lacuna

Layers of
cementum

Lacuna

Figure 60. A photomicrograph of an area of cementum seen with a higher power objective than the one used for Figure 59. Notice the canaliculi leading from the lacunae; and notice that they often are directed chiefly toward the outside surface of the root (to the right). The layer upon layer formation of cementum is clear.

of tooth root which have been resorbed following injury. While normal vertical pressures or light lateral pressures do not result in damage to the tooth root, a severe lateral pressure on a tooth may result not only in resorption of the bone of the tooth socket, but also in a localized resorption of the tooth root. Underlying dentin, as well as cementum, may be resorbed in some cases. When the cause of the resorption is removed, if the damage has not been too extensive, new cementum may be laid down over the damaged area, replacing both the lost cementum and the lost dentin.

The presence of cementoid on the outer surface of the root is an important factor in the clinical success of orthodontic treatment. Cementoid, because it is only slightly calcified, undergoes resorption less readily than bone. When the orthodontist establishes continued light lateral pressure on a tooth by the use of orthodontic appliances, the pressure is transmitted to the periodontal ligament and to the bone of the tooth socket, and the bone, not the tooth root, is resorbed. On the opposite side of the tooth socket, where the periodontal ligament is under tension (pull) due to this lateral movement, addition of bone takes place, and there is thereby an actual change in the location of the tooth socket and in the position of the tooth (Chapter 8). The difference between the pressure used by the orthodontist and the pressure which causes damage to the tooth root lies chiefly in the difference in the severity of the pressure.

Cementum is sometimes formed in excessive amounts. Excessive cementum is variously called *hypercementosis, excementosis,* or *cementum hyperplasia.* It may occur on all or on only a few of the teeth in any mouth; and it may occur over the entire tooth root or only in localized areas (Fig. 55). The causes of excessive cementum formation are not fully known. A large amount of cementum sometimes is useful in that it may furnish additional attachment for periodontal ligament fibers. Again, it may be a handicap. If it occurs as a spicule protruding from the side of the root and interlocking in a resorbed area of the lamina dura (the bone of the tooth socket), or if it occurs as excessive cementum at the root apex producing a ball-shaped root end (Fig. 61), it may create a problem in extraction if for any reason the tooth must be removed.

Cementicles are small bodies of cementum which are sometimes found in the periodontal ligament. They are usually regarded as of no clinical importance.

Mamelons

Hypercementosis

Figure 61. A photomicrograph (low power) of a ground section of a mandibular incisor tooth cut mesiodistally. Before this tooth was cut the apical half of the root looked like a round ball on the end of the tooth. This is hypercementosis. Notice, also, the conspicuous mamelons, and the pit between the left and center mamelon.

CHAPTER 7

Periodontal Ligament

(Periodontal Membrane)

LOCATION

The periodontal ligament (peri = around; odontos = tooth) is a layer of connective tissue usually less than 0.25 mm. in width which surrounds the root of a tooth, occupying the space between the tooth root and the bone of the tooth socket (Figs. 62, 66, and 76). The periodontal ligament is also called *periodontal membrane*.

STRUCTURE OF THE PERIODONTAL LIGAMENT

The periodontal ligament is made up of cells and of amorphous and fibrous intercellular substance. The most outstanding constituent is the fibrous intercellular substance which makes up the *fibers* of the periodontal ligament. Among these fibers are located *fibroblast cells, blood vessels, lymph vessels, nerves,* and in some areas small groups or strings of *epithelial cells,* and sometimes *cementicles.* In addition to these structures there are often specialized cells which function in the formation of cementum (cementoblasts) and of bone (osteoblasts); and sometimes there are specialized cells associated with the resorption of cementum (cementoclasts) and of bone (osteoclasts).

In width the periodontal ligament has been found to range from 0.12 to 0.33 mm. The width varies on different teeth and in different areas around the same tooth. Decreased function of the tooth seems to be accompanied by decreased width of the periodontal ligament.

Bundles of periodontal ligament fibers are attached at one side of the periodontal ligament to the cementum covering the tooth root; and with the exception of certain fibers around the cervix of the tooth they are attached at the other side of the periodontal ligament to the bone of the tooth socket (Fig. 62). This attachment takes place when the cementum and the bone are forming: ends of bundles of the periodontal ligament fibers become entrapped in the forming hard tissue. This attachment serves to hold the tooth firmly in the jaw. These attached heavy fiber bundles of the periodontal ligament are referred to collectively as *Sharpey's fibers* (Figs. 63 and 64).

While large bundles of fibers are attached to both cementum and bone, it does not thereby follow that each fiber of each bundle necessarily extends uninterrupted from cementum to bone. As a matter of fact, the individual fibers extend from the cementum or from the bone toward the center of the periodontal ligament where possibly some or all of them terminate, their ends being

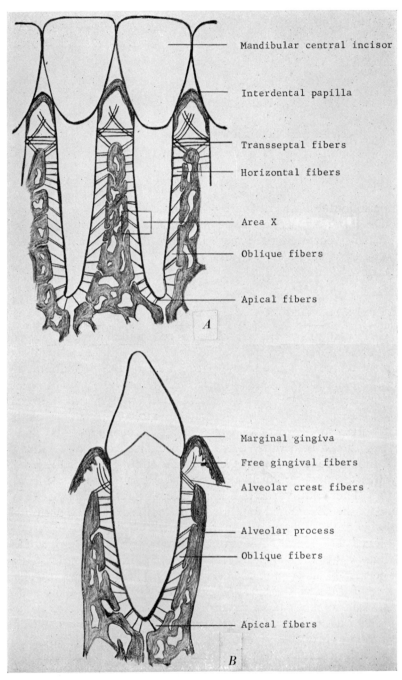

Figure 62. A diagrammatic illustration of the arrangement of the periodontal ligament fibers around the tooth roots of the mandibular incisors. The width of the periodontal ligament is exaggerated in order to show the direction of the fibers. A. Facial view. B. Proximal view. Area X in Figure A is shown in detail in Figure 63. (Adapted from Noyes, Schour, Noyes.)

interwoven with ends of fibers from the opposite direction. This area of apparently interwoven fibers is called the *intermediate plexus*. The fact that the fiber bundles seem to be spliced in the center of the periodontal ligament is is said to enable a readjustment of these fibers as a tooth moves occlusally in eruption. This statement is open to question.

Around a nonfunctioning tooth (one which is not in occlusion with the

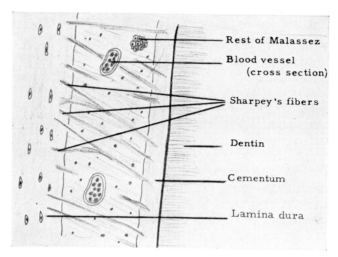

Figure 63. Diagrammatic drawing of a small area of periodontal ligament showing Sharpey's fibers. Enlargement of area X in Figure 62A.

Figure 64. A photomicrograph of an area of bone in which numerous bundles of periodontal ligament fibers are embedded. The embedded ends of these fiber bundles are known as *Sharpey's fibers*. As seen here the strength of this attachment is impressive. (High power magnification.)

teeth in the opposing arch) the periodontal ligament fibers are relaxed and wavy, with no definite orientation (Fig. 72); but around a tooth which is in heavy function the fiber bundles are stretched straight and have a characteristic orientation on different areas of the tooth root. These large, well-oriented bundles of fibers are referred to as the *principal fibers of the periodontal ligament.*

PRINCIPAL FIBERS OF THE PERIODONTAL LIGAMENT

The principal fibers of the periodontal ligament around a heavily functioning tooth have such a clear and consistent arrangement that they have been described as being composed of six groups of fibers, each group being named according to its location and orientation: (1) the *free gingival fibers,* (2) the *transseptal fibers,* (3) the *alveolar crest fibers,* (4) the *horizontal fibers,* (5) the *oblique fibers,* and (6) the *apical fibers.* Study the position of these groups of fibers in Figure 62A and B as you read their description in the text.

1. *Free gingival fibers* are located around the cervical part of the root. Bundles of these fibers are embedded at one end in the cementum. The fibers extend from the cementum out into the gingiva which surrounds the neck of the tooth. In the gingiva the heavy bundles of fibers separate into individual fibers and intermingle with the connective tissue fibers of the gingiva. Examine Figures 62A and 93 for the location and arrangement of the free gingival fibers. Notice that a pressure applied on the incisal (or occlusal) part of the tooth would cause the free gingival fibers to be stretched taut with the result that this group of fibers would function to hold the gingiva firmly to the tooth surface.

2. *Transseptal fibers* are located just apical to the gingival fiber group and are on the mesial and distal sides of the tooth only. Bundles of these fibers are embedded at one end in the cementum of one tooth and at the other end in the cementum of the adjacent tooth. With the exception of the maxillary and mandibular central incisors, where the mesial sides of the right and left centrals are connected by these fibers, the transseptal fibers extend from the cementum on the mesial side of one tooth to the cementum on the distal side of the adjacent tooth. Notice in Figure 62A how they cross over the top of the bone between the teeth. These fibers help to maintain the teeth in their proper relationship to one another.

3. *Alveolar crest fibers* are located at the level of the alveolar crest (the margin of the bone which surrounds the tooth root). These fiber bundles are embedded on one side of the periodontal ligament in the cementum of the tooth root and on the other side of the periodontal ligament in the alveolar crest. They are of course found all around the tooth. Examine Figure 62A and B and notice how the arrangement of this group of fibers helps to resist horizontal movements of the tooth.

4. *Horizontal fibers* are located apical to the alveolar crest fibers. They are embedded in the cementum of the tooth root and in the bone of the tooth socket. They lie in a horizontal position relative to the jaw bone. They are of course all around the tooth root. Examine the arrangement of these fibers in Figure 62A and you will see how they function to resist horizontal pressures applied to the tooth crown.

5. *Oblique fibers* are located immediately apical to the horizontal group of fibers. They are attached to the cementum and to the bone of the tooth socket and they run in an oblique, or diagonal, direction. Look at the orientation of these fibers in Figure 62*A* and *B*: the end attached to the bone is always more toward the tooth crown than is the end attached to the cementum. Imagine a pressure applied vertically to the incisal (or occlusal) surface of the tooth. Such a pressure would stretch the oblique fibers taut and the tooth would be literally suspended in its socket (Fig. 65). The result of such vertical pressure is a pull on, rather than a pressure on, both the cementum of the tooth root and the bone of the alveolus (tooth socket). This pull (tension) is fortunate, because continued pressure on bone ordinarily results in bone resorption. This group of strong oblique fiber bundles prevents the apex of the root from being jammed against the bottom of the socket.

At the transition between the oblique fibers and the radiating apical fibers there is a small region in which the fibers again extend in a horizontal plane. Although these fibers are usually not named in the arbitrary classification which has been given to the periodontal ligament fibers, they function with the previously described horizontal fibers in stabilizing the tooth.

6. *Apical fibers* radiate around the apex of the tooth. At approximately right angles to their attachment in the cementum they extend to their at-

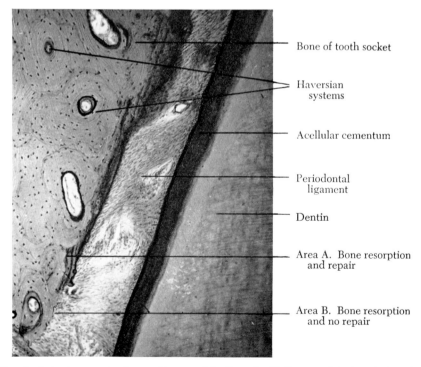

Bone of tooth socket

Haversian systems

Acellular cementum

Periodontal ligament

Dentin

Area A. Bone resorption and repair

Area B. Bone resorption and no repair

Figure 65. A photomicrograph of a small area of tooth root with the associated periodontal ligament and lamina dura. The direction of the periodontal ligament fibers shows that the crown of the tooth was at the bottom of the pictured area. Notice the resorption of the alveolar bone at area B. At area A there has been bone resorption as far as the end of the pointer line; and then there was bone apposition (addition) on the surface of the resorbed area (repair).

tachment in the bone at the base of the alveolus. As you can see by examining Figure 62A and B these apical fibers resist any force tending to lift the tooth from the socket, and function with the fibers of other groups to stabilize the tooth against forces tending to produce a tilting movement.

Scattered among the principal fibers of the periodontal ligament are other smaller fibers which have no distinct orientation.

STRUCTURES IN THE PERIODONTAL LIGAMENT

Blood vessels of the periodontal ligament are branches of the superior or the inferior alveolar artery and vein. They enter the periodontal ligament at various locations: (1) at the fundus (bottom) of the alveolus, along with vessels which supply the tooth pulp; (2) through openings in the bone of the sides of the alveolus, coming from the bone marrow spaces; and (3) from the deeper branches of gingival blood vessels which pass over the alveolar crest.

Lymphatic vessels follow the path of the blood vessels.

Nerves of the periodontal ligament generally follow the blood vessels. They are sensory nerves from the second division (in the maxilla) or the third division (in the mandible) of the fifth cranial nerve. They provide a sense of touch—that is, they enable the individual to be aware of a touch or tap given to the tooth.

Rests of Malassez are small groups of epithelial cells which are seen in microscopic examination of the periodontal ligament (Figs. 63, 94 and 96). They are sometimes called *epithelial rests*. At times such epithelial cells are seen microscopically as strings of cells rather than as round groups of cells in the periodontal ligament, in which case they are referred to as remains of *Hertwig's epithelial root sheath* (Fig. 94B).* Whatever name is applied to these epithelial cells found in the periodontal ligament, they have come to be recognized as cells derived from the enamel organ which produced the tooth enamel at the time the tooth was forming (Chapter 11). Their presence may be important pathologically in the formation of certain tumors and cyst linings.

Cementicles are minute calcified bodies sometimes seen in microscopic examination of the periodontal ligament of older individuals. Cementicles may be attached to the cementum, or they may be entirely separate from the tooth root. Their size varies but their shape is ordinarily spherical. Usually they are not considered to be of clinical importance.

Osteoblasts (osteo = bone; blast = germ) are specialized connective tissue cells which are found at the surface of bone in locations where bone formation is occurring. They may be seen in the periodontal ligament at the surface of the bone of the tooth socket in locations where bone is being laid down. *Osteoclasts* (clast = break) are specialized connective tissue cells which border bone which is being resorbed. They may occur in the periodontal ligament next to the bone of the tooth socket in locations where bone resorption is taking place. Similarly, *cementoblasts* are specialized connective tissue cells which accompany cementum formation, and *cementoclasts* are specialized connective

* Interesting paper: Valderhaug, J. and H. A. Zander: Relationship of "Epithelial Rests of Malassez" to Other Periodontal Structures, Periodontics 5:254, 1967.

tissue cells which accompany cementum resorption. These cells occur in the periodontal ligament at the surface of the cementum where cementum formation or cementum resorption is taking place. See Figure 72.

Functions and Clinical Importance of the Periodontal Ligament

The functions of the periodontal ligament may be described under five headings: (1) supportive, (2) formative, (3) resorptive, (4) sensory, and (5) nutritive.

The *supportive function* of the periodontal ligament results from the ingenious arrangement of its principal fibers. As you have seen, the fibers are so arranged that functional pressure on the tooth crown from any direction produces a tension (pulling) of certain fiber groups. Consequently, pressure on the tooth crown is transmitted to the bone of the tooth socket and to the cementum as a pull. Due to this fiber arrangement which suspends the tooth in its socket the tooth is not pressed against the bone of the socket wall during the process of biting and chewing. These sturdy principal fibers of the periodontal ligament which separate the cementum of the tooth root from the wall of the socket by less than $\frac{1}{4}$ mm. are able to withstand the tremendous force produced by the powerful jaw muscles in closing the jaws. It has been reported that the maximum biting force between the molar teeth in a group of Alaskan Eskimo men was about 348 pounds.*

A sudden excessive pressure applied to a tooth crown, such as in case of an accidental blow, may damage the periodontal ligament sufficiently to loosen the tooth.

The *formative function* of the periodontal ligament is seen in both the developing tooth and in the adult functioning tooth. During tooth development the periodontal ligament produces both the cementum of the tooth root and the bone of the tooth socket. In the functioning tooth the periodontal ligament is able to produce cementum at any time during the life of the tooth; and it maintains the bone of the tooth socket by producing new bone following bone resorption (Fig. 65).

The *resorptive function* of the periodontal ligament accompanies the formative function. Whereas tension (pull) on the periodontal ligament fibers tends to stimulate cementum and bone formation, pressure stimulates bone resorption. Severe pressure produces rapid bone resorption, and sometimes may cause resorption of the more resistant cementum as well. If sufficiently severe, pressure may destroy areas of the periodontal ligament. More will be learned about the processes of bone formation and bone resorption in the discussion of bone and the alveolar process (Chapter 8).

The *sensory function* of the periodontal ligament is seen in the ability of an individual to estimate the amount of pressure in mastication and to identify which one of several teeth receives a slight tap with an instrument.

The *nutritive function* is served by the presence of blood vessels in the periodontal ligament.

It is obvious that without the periodontal ligament a tooth cannot be retained in its socket. Localized destruction of the periodontal ligament may

* Waugh, L. M.: Jour. Dent. Res., *16*:355, 1937.

be repaired by the formation of new tissue when the cause of the destruction is removed. Localized detachment from the cementum of the principal fibers of the periodontal ligament may be followed by fiber reattachment if removal of irritating factors permits the formation of new cementum. Extensive destruction of the periodontal ligament may result in the necessity for the removal of the tooth.

CHAPTER 8

Bone and the Alveolar* Process

BONE

The word *bone* is used to designate both a tissue and an organ. *Bone*, a tissue, is one of the connective tissues. It is made up of (1) an organic matrix which calcifies and (2) osteocytes (bone cells). *A bone*, an organ, such as the mandible, for example, is composed of bone tissue; it contains in its center bone marrow, and it has closely associated with it blood vessels and nerves.

GROSS STRUCTURE OF A BONE (an organ)

Bones are solid-looking organs, but they are not solid structures throughout. The bone tissue of which bones are composed may be described in two classes: (1) *compact bone* and (2) *trabecular bone* (or *cancellous bone*). The outside wall of a bone, the mandible, for example, is compact bone; but the mandible has a hollow center, the *bone marrow cavity*, into which *trabeculae* (bars or plates) of bone protrude. These trabeculae make up trabecular bone. In the spaces around the trabeculae in the bone marrow cavity is the *bone marrow*.

Examine Figure 66 which is a drawing of a cross section of a human mandible, and Figure 76 which is a drawing of a longitudinal section of a human mandible. Notice the compact character of the bone which makes up the outer wall of the mandible and the trabeculae which project into the marrow cavity. The number and size of the trabeculae in the marrow cavity of a bone are determined to a large degree by the functional activity of the organ: the greater the functional activity the greater the number of trabeculae.

Certain advantages result from this arrangement of bone tissue into compact and trabecular bone. For one thing, a large bone with trabeculae and bone marrow in its center is much lighter in weight than would be the same organ composed of solid bone tissue throughout. Also, the presence of the bone marrow makes available to the bone tissue nutrition from blood vessels which are located inside the organ as well as from blood vessels which lie on the outside surface.

The outside surface of all bones is covered by a thin connective tissue membrane called the *periosteum* (peri = around; osteum = bone). The inside surfaces of bones are covered with a much more delicate connective tissue membrane called the *endosteum* (endo = within) (Fig. 66).

* Pronounced ăl vē′ ō lĕr.

— Tooth

— Calculus
— Epithelial attachment

— Inflammation in gingiva

Intact alveolar crest

Resorption of alveolar crest

Periodontal ligament

Cortical plate
                            } Alveolar
Trabecular bone {   process
Lamina dura

Location of endosteum

Mental foramen

Location of periosteum

Genioglossus
muscle

Bone marrow cavity

Salivary gland
Geniohyoid muscle

Mylohyoid muscle

Digastric muscle
(anterior belly)

Figure 66. Diagrammatic drawing of a faciolingual section of a human mandible in the region of the second premolar tooth (much enlarged). This section is not cut through the pulp cavity of the tooth.

Periosteum
Circumferential lamellae
Volkmann's canal

Haversian canal (X section)
Haversian lamellae

Figure 67. Photomicrograph of a ground cross section of human femur. (Low power magnification.) At the top of the picture is the bone surface with a portion of the periosteum still adhering to it in some places. The bone lamellae at the surface have a circumferential arrangement. Beneath the circumferential lamellae are Haversian systems where the lamellae are in concentric layers. In the center of each Haversian system is the Haversian canal. In several places a Volkmann's canal enters an Haversian canal. Near the bottom of the picture Volkmann's canals are entering an Haversian canal from two directions. In the upper right two Volkmann's canals enter from the outside of the organ. The one marked x is seen in higher magnification in Figure 68.

MICROSCOPIC STRUCTURE OF BONE (a tissue)

Bone tissue consists of bone cells and a bone matrix which is made up of two kinds of intercellular substance, fibrous and amorphous. The intercellular substance becomes calcified, which makes bone a hard tissue. Bone is about 50 per cent mineral substance and about 50 per cent organic substance. It has about the same hardness as cementum.

The cells of bone tissue, *osteocytes* (osteo = bone; cyte = cell), are distributed throughout the calcified intercellular substance. The space in the bone matrix which is occupied by an osteocyte is called a *lacuna* (little space) (Figs. 68 and 69). Lacunae are connected with one another by a system of *canaliculi* (little canals). These canaliculi extend not only from one lacuna to another, but some of them open into the various canals of bone where capillaries are located. Tissue fluids pass from the capillaries to the canaliculi and hence from one lacuna to another throughout the bone tissue.

Mature bone tissue is formed in thin layers, called *lamellae*. These lamellae have two different patterns of arrangement, and according to their pattern bone tissue is called either *Haversian system bone* or *lamellar bone*.

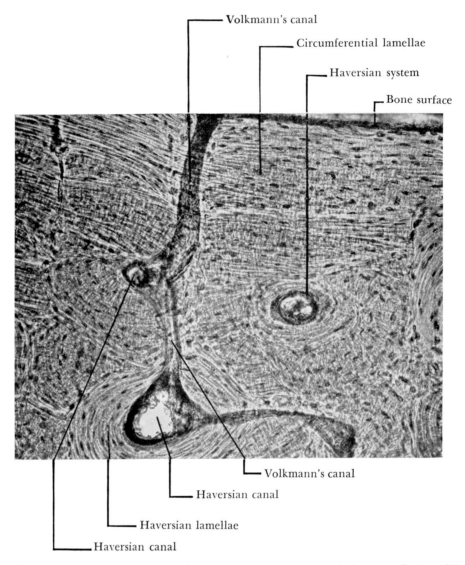

Volkmann's canal

Circumferential lamellae

Haversian system

Bone surface

Volkmann's canal

Haversian canal

Haversian lamellae

Haversian canal

Figure 68. This photomicrograph of a ground section of bone is a higher magnification of the area marked x in Figure 67. The surface of the bone is seen in the upper right. A Volkmann's canal cuts through the surface circumferential lamellae and enters an Haversian canal slightly at left of center. The Volkmann's canal continues (toward bottom of picture) to a second Haversian canal (note the concentric bone lamellae around the canal). The Volkmann's canal then turns right (across bottom of picture). By such a route blood vessels and nerves supply bone tissue.

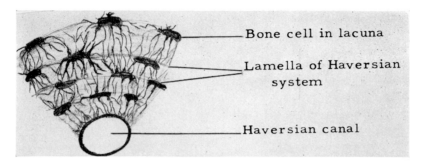

Bone cell in lacuna

Lamella of Haversian system

Haversian canal

Figure 69. Diagrammatic drawing of a sector of an Haversian system cut in cross section. This is greatly enlarged. The diameter of an Haversian system is something more or less than 0.1 mm.

In *Haversian system bone* the lamellae are arranged in concentric circles around a very small central canal which is called an *Haversian canal*. A series of concentric lamellae with the included Haversian canal is called an *Haversian system* (Figs. 67, 68, and 69). An Haversian system may have from 4 to 20 concentric lamellae and may measure somewhat more or less than 0.1 mm. in diameter.

In *lamellar bone* the lamellae are not arranged in small concentric circles. Lamellar bone makes up the outside surface of most bones, the lamellae following the surface, or circumference, of the bone (Figs. 67 and 68). In this location the lamellar bone is sometimes given the additional names of *circumferential bone*, or *subperiosteal bone* (subperiosteal = beneath the periosteum). Lamellar bone also often makes up the surfaces of the trabeculae of trabecular bone; and in this location it may be called *subendosteal bone* (beneath the endosteum). Both patterns of arrangement of lamellae, *i.e.*, Haversian system bone and lamellar bone, are found in all mature human bone.

Regardless of the arrangement of bone lamellae, bone tissue contains osteocytes which lie in lacunae and connect through canaliculi. This system of connected bone cells (Fig. 69) is the means by which nutrients are distributed throughout the bone tissue. In an Haversian system some of the canaliculi open into the Haversian canal, providing a pathway by which nutrients from the blood vessels contained in the canal may reach the osteocytes of the Haversian system.

Bone is a very vascular tissue; it contains many blood vessels. Arteries and veins enter and leave a bone in various places both from the outside surface and from the bone marrow cavity. The canals in a bone through which blood vessels pass into the bone tissue from the outside of the organ or from the bone marrow cavity are called *Volkmann's canals* (Figs. 67 and 68). Branches of the blood vessels contained in Volkmann's canals enter the smaller Haversian canals.

It seems remarkable that blood vessels should enter bones and be distributed throughout bones in the way that they are; but actually, in the embryonic development of the body, the larger blood vessels are formed and are in place before bone formation begins. As bone is formed it simply surrounds and encloses any blood vessels located in the area. Therefore we find blood vessels entering and leaving bones at various points.

Bone marrow, which occupies the centers of bones in the spaces around the trabeculae, is a soft tissue (Figs. 66 and 76). There are two types of bone marrow: (1) *red marrow,* which is found in most of the bones of young individuals and has the function of producing red and white blood cells; and (2) *yellow marrow* (fat marrow), which does not have a blood-forming function. In adults most red marrow becomes converted into yellow marrow. Only certain locations in the adult skeleton retain the red type of marrow which continues to perform the function of hemopoiesis (hemo = blood; poiesis = creation).

Periosteum and Endosteum

On the outside surface a bone is covered by a more or less tough connective tissue membrane called the *periosteum.* A thinner, more delicate connective tissue membrane, called the *endosteum,* covers the inner surface of compact bone and the trabeculae in the bone marrow cavity, and lines the Haversian canals and the Volkmann's canals. These two membranes, the periosteum and the endosteum, function both in the formation and in the resorption of bone tissue.

The periodontal ligament which surrounds the root of a tooth and separates it from the bone of the tooth socket is a specialized periosteum. It functions on one side in the formation and resorption of the bone comprising the tooth socket and on the other side in the formation and resorption of the cementum covering the tooth root.

Growth of Bone

Bone growth includes both *bone formation* and *bone resorption.*

Bone formation is the conversion of relatively unspecialized connective tissue into bone matrix and bone cells, and the subsequent calcification of the bone matrix. Bone matrix is composed of two kinds of intercellular substance: fibrous and amorphous. It arises as a result of a chemical change which takes place in the fibrous and amorphous intercellular substances of unspecialized connective tissue. The bone cells are certain cells of this same connective tissue which are entrapped in the forming bone matrix. In a growing bone the connective tissue which forms the new bone is the periosteum, or the endosteum, as the case may be, depending on whether the new bone is being added to the outside or to the inside of the organ. The intercellular substance of the part of the periosteum (or endosteum) which lies against the bone surface is chemically changed into bone matrix. Some of the cells of the periosteum (or endosteum) next to the bone surface become specialized and are called *osteoblasts* (osteo = bone; blast = germ) (Figs. 71 and 72). As the new bone matrix is formed, some of these osteoblasts become surrounded by it and so become cells of the bone tissue, *osteocytes.* Because the osteoblasts in the periosteum (or endosteum) are not completely isolated cells but have their cytoplasm connected with other osteoblasts by numerous thin projections, the osteocytes likewise are not isolated cells but have their cytoplasm connected with other osteocytes by the same thin projections (Fig. 69). The spaces in the bone matrix occupied by the osteocytes are the lacunae; and the spaces occupied by the numerous cytoplasmic connections are the canaliculi.

In the embryonic development of certain bones the formation of bone tissue is preceded by the formation of a cartilage structure which resembles in shape the bone that is to be formed and which serves as a pattern for the future bone. This cartilage predecessor of the bone calcifies and then is gradually removed by resorption. As the calcified cartilage is resorbed, bone tissue is formed to replace it. Bones which arise in this way, with a cartilage structure preceding the development of bone tissue, are said to be formed by *endochondral formation*. Examples of bones formed in this manner are the long bones of the arms and legs.

In the embryonic development of other bones, the bone tissue is formed without a preceding cartilage pattern, and these bones are said to be formed by *intramembranous formation* (Fig. 70). Examples of bones formed in this manner, with no preceding cartilage structure, are the mandible and the maxillae. The process of the conversion of unspecialized connective tissue into bone and the final microscopic structure of bone tissue are the same whether or not bone formation has been preceded by cartilage.

At first glance bone appears to be a permanent and unchanging tissue. Actually, bone is in a state of constant change. Bone tissue formation continues practically throughout the life of the bone, but the organ does not thereby become indefinitely heavier and greater in mass. The density and size of a bone are limited by the fact that the formation of bone tissue in one place is compensated for by the resorption of bone tissue in another.

New bone

Osteoblasts in area of bone formation

Figure 70. A photomicrograph of a section of forming bone in the area of the mandible in a kitten fetus. This is intramembranous bone formation. Osteoblasts are numerous. The connective tissue from which the bone is forming is in the lower right corner. (Medium power magnification.)

Bone resorption is the removal of both the mineral materials and the organic matrix of bone. Resorption of bone should not be confused with decalcification of bone (or other hard tissues) such as occurs when the tissue is removed from the body and taken to the laboratory to be placed in a weak acid solution. In this laboratory procedure, called decalcification, the mineral material is removed and the organic material remains. In bone resorption, the organic matrix and the mineral material are both removed, and nothing of the bone remains.

Bone resorption occurs just beneath the periosteum or endosteum. A specialized type of cell called an *osteoclast* (clast = break) is associated with the resorption of bone tissue (Fig. 73). Osteoclasts are multinucleated cells (contain more than one nucleus), the nuclei ranging from 2 or 3 to a dozen or more in a single cell. Osteoclasts, like osteoblasts, originate from the cells of the periosteum or endosteum. Their function is not clearly understood, but their presence, seen microscopically, is an indication that bone resorption was occurring in this tissue (Figs. 71 and 72).

Bone formation and bone resorption are processes that occur intermittently in all bones throughout the life of the individual. The intramembranous bone (Fig. 70) and the endochondral bone that form in the early development of the individual are gradually resorbed and are replaced by mature bone. With growth and function the mature bone undergoes an endless process of resorp-

Bone

Osteoclast
(bone resorption)

Osteoblasts
(bone formation)

Enamel organ of
a developing tooth

Figure 71. A photomicrograph of a small area of kitten mandible in the region of developing teeth. The large triangular piece of bone shows bone resorption on one side (*left*) and bone formation on the other side (*right*). In the area of bone resorption are a large number of osteoclasts on the bone surface. Resorption in this area is probably due to the presence of a developing tooth, the enamel organ of which is seen in the lower left. On the right side of the triangular bone the presence of numerous, closely packed osteoblasts on the bone surface are associated with formation of bone tissue in this area. (Low power magnification.)

Cementum on
tooth root

Periodontal
ligament

Bone

Osteoclast in
area of bone
resorption

Osteoblasts in
area of bone
formation

Figure 72. A photomicrograph of an area of tooth root, periodontal ligament, and alveolar bone (lamina dura). This was a tooth not in function: notice the lack of orientation of periodontal ligament fibers. There is bone resorption on the bone surface next to the periodontal ligament. Notice the osteoclasts. On the other surface of the bone (to the right) the presence of osteoblasts indicates bone formation. (Medium power magnification.)

Bone

Osteoclast

Figure 73. A photomicrograph (high power magnification) of osteoclasts in the area of bone development of a kitten mandible. Bone development of course includes bone resorption as well as bone formation and the presence of osteoclasts indicates that this is an area of resorption. Bone is at the top of the picture; bone-forming connective tissue is at the bottom. The osteoclast in the center of the picture distinctly shows the presence of nine nuclei.

tion in one place and apposition (formation) in another. Haversian systems are partially or wholly resorbed and then replaced by other Haversian systems or by lamellar bone. Lamellar bone is resorbed and replaced by Haversian system bone or by new lamellar bone. This turnover is rapid during the growth of the individual, and occurs more slowly later in life. After full individual growth is attained, however, the processes of bone change may occur rapidly in places where function or trauma stimulate resorption or apposition.

Bone formation and bone resorption are taking place almost continuously in some areas of the bone tissue that surrounds the teeth. They occur in response to certain stimuli. In the tooth socket the stimuli which govern bone formation and bone resorption are: (1) tension (pull) on the periodontal ligament fibers attached to the bone, and (2) pressure on the periodontal ligament and on the bone. Tension on the periodontal ligament fibers induces bone formation; pressure induces bone resorption.

THE ALVEOLAR PROCESS

The *alveolar process* is defined as that part of the mandible and maxillae which surrounds and supports the teeth (Fig. 74). The alveolar process supports the tooth roots on the facial and on the palatal and lingual sides; it extends between the teeth, separating them on the mesial and distal sides; and it extends into the furcation of the roots of multirooted teeth (Figs. 66 and 76). The occlusal border of the alveolar process, located near the cervix of the tooth, is referred to as the *alveolar crest*.

Figure 74. A human maxilla. The palatal part of the alveolar process merges without a distinct line into the bone of the palate. The alveolar process extending between the teeth is seen clearly. The alveolar crest is the edge of the alveolar process around the cervix of the tooth. Notice the attrition of the incisal edges of the anterior teeth.

The alveolar process may be described as being composed of the *lamina dura** and the *supporting bone*. The lamina dura is the bone of the wall of the tooth socket. The supporting bone is made up of (1) the *cortical plate*, which is the outside wall of the mandible and the maxillae and (2) the *trabecular bone* which is located between the lamina dura and the cortical bone in many areas (Figs. 66, 74, 75, 76, and 93). In some areas the alveolar process is thin and contains little or no trabecular bone: the lamina dura and the cortical plate are fused. This kind of thin alveolar process is found, among other places, on the facial surfaces of mandibular anterior teeth.

CLINICAL ASPECTS OF BONE REACTION IN THE ALVEOLAR PROCESS

The trabecular bone and the lamina dura which support a tooth react in different ways to changes in tooth function. When a tooth is in strong masticatory function, the trabecular bone in the alveolar process and the trabecular bone beneath the alveolus† of the tooth are composed of numerous heavy bone trabeculae. If the tooth is removed from function by loss of opposing teeth, these supporting trabeculae become less numerous and smaller. If the tooth in question is again placed in occlusion by the replacement of the lost teeth in the opposing arch, more trabecular bone will again form around the tooth which has resumed masticatory function.

The lamina dura, which comprises the tooth socket, does not respond by resorption to loss of masticatory function of the tooth. However, the lamina dura may respond by resorption to various stimuli such as trauma due to faulty occlusion, or periodontal disease, or pressures produced during orthodontic treatment, or pressures produced by mesial drift (see Chapter 12). Also, addition of bone tissue to the lamina dura at the base of the alveolus may be a factor in the continued occlusal movement of a tooth as attrition on the occlusal or incisal surface takes place. This addition to the lamina dura and the addition of cementum to the root, may partially compensate for loss of crown length due to attrition.

Inflammation and swelling of the soft tissues around a tooth may result in damage to the periodontal ligament and resorption of the crest of the alveolar process (Figs. 66 and 96). The presence of calculus in the gingival sulcus has the potentiality to set off a series of events: The calculus produces inflammation and swelling of the adjacent soft tissues. This condition involves and damages the periodontal ligament fibers around the neck of the tooth. Damage to the periodontal ligament results in resorption of the bone to which the fibers are attached. Continued inflammation produces continued bone resorption. Eventually so much damage may be done to the periodontal ligament and to the lamina dura that removal of the tooth becomes necessary.

Good oral hygiene and prompt dental care will prevent such serious involvement because of the following consequential reactions: (1) Removal of the calculus may be expected to result in the elimination of the inflammation and swelling. (2) Elimination of the inflammation and swelling permits repair of the periodontal ligament. (3) At the same time there will be an arrest of

---

* Also called *alveolar bone, true alveolar bone, alveolar bone proper*, and *cribriform plate*.
† Pronounced *ăl vē′ ō lŭs* (the tooth socket).

8

Maxillary third molar

Trabecular bone

Mandibular third molar

Figure 75. A human maxilla and mandible with the facial parts of the alveolar process removed excepting near the cervical border. In the mandible some trabecular bone remains among the tooth roots. Notice the location and position of the developing mandibular and maxillary third molars. (Chapters 11 and 12.) The crown of the mandibular third molar is nearly completed in the ramus of the mandible. Its occlusal surface is directed mesially and occlusally. It is surrounded by a bony crypt. The maxillary third molar is directed buccally and distally.

Figure 76. Diagrammatic drawing of a section of a human mandible bearing an isolated first molar tooth, cut mesiodistally. 1. Pulp horn. 2. Gingival fibers of periodontal ligament. 3. Bone of interradicular septum (between the roots). 4. Cortical bone on ridge of mandible. 5. Lamina dura bone near apex of distal root. 6. Cross section small blood vessel. 7. Fat marrow. 8. Trabecular bone scattered throughout bone marrow cavity. 9. Longitudinal section blood vessel. 10. Inferior alveolar nerve. 11. Cortical bone on inferior surface of mandible. A, B, C, and D indicate different areas of the periodontal ligament. A, the periodontal ligament on the mesial side of the mesial root; and B, the periodontal ligament on the mesial side of the distal root. At both A and B the principal fibers have a wavy appearance and there is evidence of resorption of the lamina dura bone. C, the periodontal ligament on the distal side of the mesial root; and D, the periodontal ligament on the distal side of the distal root. At C and D the principal fibers are straight and there is no evidence of resorption of the lamina dura. It may be inferred that this tooth was undergoing a slight movement in a mesial direction: the slight pressure on the mesial side of each root resulted in relaxed periodontal ligament fibers and in bone resorption in the lamina dura. On the distal side of each root the fibers are straight and there is no evidence of bone resorption.

Figure 76. *Legend on opposite page.*

the resorption of the bone of the alveolar crest. (4) Additional cementum may be produced on the tooth root in the affected area with an accompanying re-attachment of the previously damaged periodontal ligament. (5) Repair of some of the resorbed areas of the lamina dura may occur, and some bone construction may possibly take place on the alveolar crest. It is probable that the alveolar crest will occupy a position apical to that of the original position— that is, there will not be enough bone replacement on the alveolar crest to make it as high as it was originally.

Teeth are sometimes, either by accident or by design, subjected to pressure on the crown from a horizontal direction (Fig. 76). If the pressure is con-tinued and is not so severe as to damage the periodontal ligament, it will produce an adaptive response in the lamina dura. On the side of the tooth socket toward which the tooth is pushed the periodontal ligament and the lamina dura are subjected to pressures, and bone resorption occurs. On the side of the tooth socket away from which the tooth is pulled the periodontal ligament fibers are subjected to tension, and additional bone of the lamina dura is formed. The result of this bone resorption and bone formation is a change in the location of the tooth socket and also, of course, in the location of the tooth.

Such a change in the position of a tooth may be a result of a change in occlusal pressures. Or it may be a consequence of treatment applied by the orthodontist to improve unsatisfactory tooth alignment. The orthodontist places appliances on a patient's teeth and adjusts them at intervals so that proper pressures and tensions are maintained. The teeth being treated actu-ally change location in the mouth. The success of this treatment is due to three factors: (1) Bone is resorbed more easily than cementum. (2) The area of the lamina dura toward which the tooth is moved is resorbed. (3) The area of the lamina dura away from which the tooth is moved is built up.

CHAPTER 9

The Oral Mucous Membrane and the Salivary Glands

MUCOUS MEMBRANES

Definition

A mucous membrane is the lining of a body cavity that opens to the outside of the body. Mucous membranes are found lining the oral cavity, the nasal cavity and sinuses, the trachea, the stomach and intestines, the urinary bladder, the uterus.

Histologic Structure of Mucous Membranes

Histologically a mucous membrane is a modified skin. It is made up of two layers: (1) a surface layer of *epithelial tissue* and (2) an underlying layer of *connective tissue*. Mucous membranes are structurally less thick and tough than the skin; and whereas the skin is kept slightly moist by secretions from oil glands and sweat glands which empty onto the surface, mucous membranes are kept very moist by secretions from mucous glands, serous glands, or other secretory cells which empty onto the surface. The epithelium of a mucous membrane is protective in function, and in some areas it is also secretory and absorptive in function. The connective tissue of a mucous membrane underlies the epithelium and contains blood vessels, nerves, and sometimes glands.

Mucous membranes in different parts of the body differ in a number of ways, and in each location their structure seems to be excellently suited to perform the functions required. In places where the mucous membrane is normally protected from wear and tear it is very thin and delicate, while in areas which are subjected to functional friction it is thicker and resistant to injury.

Protected cavities such as the nasal cavity, the stomach, and the intestines are lined by delicate types of mucous membranes. *In the nasal cavity* the epithelial part of the mucous membrane is composed of pseudostratified columnar cells (Fig. 10*D*). Many of these columnar cells have *cilia*—tiny hair-like projections—on their exposed ends, while others, called *goblet cells*, secrete mucus which keeps the surface of the mucosa moist. The connective tissue part of the nasal mucous membrane is likewise thin and delicate, and contains nerves and blood vessels, and mucous and serous glands which open onto the surface of the mucosa. This moist, ciliated mucous membrane of the nasal passage functions as a dirt-catcher and helps to prevent the dust which is inhaled with the air from reaching the lungs.

Lining the stomach is a mucous membrane which is somewhat thicker than that of the nasal cavity, and which is arranged in many folds and wrinkles. The epithelium of the stomach mucosa is made up of simple columnar cells which are without cilia and which have a secretory function. The underlying connective tissue contains many glands.

In many respects resembling the stomach mucosa, the *mucosa of the small intestine* has an epithelium composed of simple columnar cells some of which are goblet cells that secrete mucus and others of which have the function of absorbing food materials from the intestine. The connective tissue contains many glands.

Contrasted with these protected, delicate mucous membranes of the nasal cavity, the stomach and the intestines is the more sturdy *mucosa which lines the oral cavity.* The lining of the mouth is constantly subjected to rubbing and scraping, not only by the process of mastication of food but also by the presence of the teeth in the mouth; and here again the structure of the mucous membrane is suited to its usage.

THE ORAL MUCOUS MEMBRANE

HISTOLOGIC STRUCTURE OF ORAL MUCOUS MEMBRANE

The mucous membrane lining the mouth is heavier and more resistant to injury than the mucous membranes of more protected cavities. Its histologic structure enables the oral mucosa to withstand the wear and tear of ordinary oral function and to resist bacterial infection. Like all mucous membranes, the oral mucosa is composed of a combination of epithelial tissue and connective tissue.

The *epithelial portion of the oral mucosa* is stratified squamous in character— that is, the epithelial cells are mostly flat in shape and are several layers deep. As in all stratified squamous epithelium, the basal layer of epithelial cells, which rests upon the connective tissue, is composed of cuboidal rather than flat cells; and it is in this basal layer that most of the cell division takes place. As new epithelial cells are produced by mitosis in the basal layer, some of the basal cells and the cells superficial to them are forced outward and eventually they reach the surface.

Different things happen to these surface epithelial cells in different parts of the mouth. In areas of the mouth where the mucosa is relatively protected, such as on the inside of the cheeks and lips and on the under side of the tongue, the surface epithelial cells are sloughed off into the saliva as new epithelial cells are produced in the basal layer (Fig. 11). A scraping from the inside of the cheeks spread onto a glass slide and examined under the microscope will be seen to contain squamous epithelial cells.

In some other parts of the mouth where the oral mucosa is subject to considerable wear and tear, such as the hard palate and the gingiva, the surface epithelial cells are not sloughed off (Fig. 77). Instead, they lose their nuclei and their cell boundaries and form a noncellular, tough, protective layer on the surface of the stratified squamous epithelial cells. This tough layer is

Keratinized
layer

Stratified
squamous
epithelium

Connective
tissue

Figure 77. A photomicrograph of a section of human gingiva.
(As seen under low power magnification.)

called the *keratin* layer*, and epithelium on which such a layer occurs is called *keratinized* epithelium*. The keratin layer wears with use, of course, but it is continuously replaced by the aging cells beneath it.

The *connective tissue portion of the oral mucosa* is composed chiefly of fibrous connective tissue in which are blood vessels and nerves. It is separated from the overlying stratified squamous epithelium by a thin basement membrane. In most places the junction between the connective tissue and the epithelium is an irregular boundary with projections of connective tissue extending like fingers up into the epithelium, but not reaching the surface. In some areas of the oral mucosa these projections are characteristically much longer and more numerous than in other areas (Figs. 11 and 77). This irregularity of contact surfaces between the two tissues serves to increase the area from which the epithelium can receive nourishment from the underlying connective tissue.

The connective tissue of the oral mucosa varies in thickness in different parts of the mouth; and it also varies in the nature of its attachment to the underlying tissue. In some areas of the mouth the connective tissue of the oral mucosa is attached firmly to underlying bone, as in the part of the gingiva which is attached to the periosteum of the alveolar process. In other areas of the mouth the connective tissue of the oral mucosa rests upon a looser

* Pronounced *kĕr′ a tĭn, kĕr′ a tĭn īzed.*

type of connective tissue called the *submucosa*, which contains larger blood vessels, nerves, glands, and fat tissue. Such an attachment of oral mucosa to submucosa is seen in the cheek. The character of the submucosa varies in different parts of the mouth, and its nature helps to determine the character of the mucosa which it supports.

For convenience in discussion an attempt has been made to classify the different areas of oral mucosa. The classification divides the oral mucosa into three categories: (1) the *masticatory mucosa*, (2) the *lining mucosa*, and (3) the *specialized mucosa*. If you will carefully examine someone's mouth and observe the mucosa in different places, such a division will seem logical.

Masticatory mucosa

Gingiva
Hard palate

Lining mucosa

Lips and cheeks
Floor of mouth
Under side of tongue
Soft palate
Alveolar mucosa

Specialized mucosa

Dorsum of tongue

The *masticatory mucosa* is the name given to the mucous membrane of the *gingiva* and of the *hard palate*. These are the areas of the oral mucosa most used during the mastication of food. The epithelium of the masticatory mucosa is usually keratinized.

Looking into a person's mouth you will see that the necks of the teeth and the bone in which the teeth are set are covered with a firm mucous membrane which fits close around the teeth and is tightly attached to the bone. This part of the oral mucosa is called the *gingiva* (Figs. 78 and 79). The gingiva is usually keratinized, is firm, and has a stippled appearance. Except for a narrow zone around the necks of the teeth the gingival mucosa is attached firmly to the underlying tissue. If you will examine the facial side of the upper and lower jaws, you will notice that several millimeters rootward from the margin of the gingiva there is a scalloped line which divides the *gingival mucosa* from the alveolar mucosa (Figs. 78 and 79). The *alveolar mucosa* may be distinguished from the gingiva because it is redder, shiny, and loose-fitting.

The mucosa covering the *hard palate* is usually well keratinized (Fig. 80). It is attached directly to the bone of the roof of the mouth only in the area of the *palatine raphe*,* which is the anteroposterior elevation in the center of the hard palate that you can feel with your tongue. On either side of the palatine raphe the palatine mucosa has a *submucosa* between it and the bone. In the anterior part the submucosa in the hard palate contains much fat

---

* Pronounced *rā′ fē*.

Figure 78. The subject of this photograph was a young woman twenty-two years old. The gingival margin fits snugly against the enamel of the tooth crowns, and the interdental papillae fill the interdental spaces (the spaces between the teeth cervical to the areas of contact). The alveolar mucosa is clearly seen in the maxillary vestibule; it is seen less clearly in this picture in the mandibular vestibule.

tissue, and in the posterior part it contains large salivary glands of the mucous type. The ducts of these glands open onto the surface of the palate mucosa. These small openings usually are not visible to the naked eye.

Notwithstanding the presence of the fat tissue and gland tissue in the submucosa of the hard palate, the oral mucosa in this area is firmly attached to the underlying bone structure. This is accomplished by strands of connective tissue which extend from the mucosa through the submucosa and attach firmly to the bone of the roof of the mouth.

Lining mucosa is located in those areas of the oral cavity where the mucous membrane might logically be regarded as functioning as a lining organ rather than as a masticatory organ. Such nonmasticatory areas are the floor of the mouth and the underside of the tongue (Fig. 81), the alveolar mucosa (Fig. 79), the soft palate, and the inside of the cheeks and lips. In none of these areas is the mucosa firmly attached to underlying bone, and ordinarily the epithelium in these areas is not keratinized.

Examine someone's mouth and ask the person to lift his tongue (Fig. 81). The floor of the mouth and the underside of the tongue are covered with lining mucosa, the epithelium of which is nonkeratinized, shiny, and thin

Figure 79. The subject is the same as in Figure 78. The line between the gingiva and the alveolar mucosa of the lower jaw is clear. Notice the loose-fitting appearance of the alveolar mucosa, and the minute blood vessels which are close to the surface. The gingiva is firm, light in color, and has a stippled (pitted) surface texture.

enough that blood vessels located in the underlying connective tissue are clearly visible. The fold of mucosa extending lengthwise in the center of the under surface of the tongue is the *lingual frenum*. Comparison of this frenum in a number of individuals will reveal that it varies considerably in size and extent. At the lower end of the lingual frenum, where the under surface of the tongue is attached to the floor of the mouth, is a nearly horizontal fold of tissue extending to the right and left of the frenum. This horizontal fold is the *plica sublingualis.** Along the crest of the plica sublingualis are small openings of ducts, usually invisible to the naked eye, which lead from the sublingual salivary glands and empty into the mouth beneath the tongue. In the center of the plica sublingualis, one on either side of the base of the lingual frenum, are the larger openings of *Wharton's ducts* which carry the salivary secretions from the submandibular glands, and also from the sublingual glands, to the oral cavity. If you have ever opened your mouth and been surprised by having two thin streams of saliva shoot out from beneath your tongue, you now know where they came from.

Now, continuing your examination of the mouth, pull the lower lip down and out and the upper lip up and out, and then pull the cheeks back at the corners of the mouth. Notice the alveolar mucosa which lines the *oral*

* Pronounced *plī' kȧ sŭb lĭng guăl' ĭs*

Figure 80. The subject is the same as in Figure 78. The hard palate is well keratinized; the palatine rugae (the horizontal ridges behind the anterior teeth) are distinct. The palatine raphe, distinguished with difficulty in this photograph, extends from anterior to posterior in the center line. Notice how the gingiva fits snugly around the palatal sides of the teeth.

Figure 81. The subject is the same as in Figure 78. This is a photograph of the floor of the mouth and part of the under surface of the elevated tongue; the mandibular anterior teeth are at the bottom of the picture. The *lingual frenum*, which tends to hold the tongue to the floor of the mouth, divides the area into right and left halves. The horizontal fold (the *sublingual fold*, or *plica sublingualis*), lying where the base of the tongue meets the floor of the mouth, bears the openings of the ducts from the sublingual and submandibular glands.

vestibules.* The epithelium of this mucosa is nonkeratinized, shiny, red, and partially transparent to underlying blood vessels. It is clearly demarcated from the paler gingival mucosa by a scalloped line (Figs. 78 and 79).

The *soft palate,* which begins about at the distal side of the maxillary third molar teeth, is a mass of flexible muscle covered on the oral surface with oral mucosa. The epithelium of this mucosa ordinarily is not keratinzed. Numerous salivary glands lie beneath the mucosa of the soft palate and empty onto its surface.

In the cheeks and lips there is a thick submucosa which contains fat tissue and also many salivary glands whose minute duct openings are scattered over the surface of the mucosa. Occasionally you may see what appears to be a pea-sized bubble just beneath the surface. This condition is due to a stoppage in one of these small salivary ducts which has resulted in an accumulation at this point of the secretion from a salivary gland. This bubble is called a *mucocele.†*

If you will examine the cheek mucosa inside the corners of the mouth of several individuals you will often find an area which has a few, or numerous, small yellowish spots which are called *Fordyce's spots.* These spots are openings onto the oral mucosa of sebaceous glands, which, of course, are usually thought of as being restricted to the skin on the outside of the body. They occur here, it is said, as a result of the narrowing of the wide embryonic mouth during early face development—*i.e.,* in the fusion of the maxillary process and the mandibular arch at either corner of the mouth some skin glands are entrapped at the line of union (Fig. 6). However near fact this explanation may be, it does not account for the presence of sebaceous glands on the red margin of the upper lip, and their usual absence on the lower lip; their presence on areas of cheek mucosa above, below, and behind the fusion line of the maxillary process and the mandibular arch; their seeming absence in human fetuses; nor their greater numbers in adults than in children.

There is an interesting bit of history connected with the observation of sebaceous glands in the oral cavity. Yellow spots in the oral mucosa were described but not recognized as sebaceous glands, in 1896 by Fordyce. Later histologists attached Fordyce's name to them, unaware of the German publication of 1862 in which these spots had been clearly described and properly identified as sebaceous glands by Kolliker. In such devious ways does man learn what he knows.‡

Specialized mucosa is the term applied to the mucous membrane located on the dorsum (top side) of the tongue. The mucosa in this area is distinctly different from other oral mucosa. Examine someone's tongue and you will see that the mucosa of its upper surface is formed into innumerable small *papillae.* These papillae are of several kinds, different in size and shape, and some of them bear microscopic organs which supply the sense of taste.

---

* The maxillary and mandibular *oral vestibules* are the spaces between the facial surfaces of the teeth and their supporting bone and the oral surfaces of the cheeks and lips. A finger inserted in the mouth between the teeth and the cheek or lip is in the *vestibule.*

† Pronounced *mū′ kô sēl.*

‡ Interesting paper: Miles, A. E. W.: Sebaceous Glands in Lip and Cheek Mucosa, Brit. Dent. Jour. *105*:235, 1958.

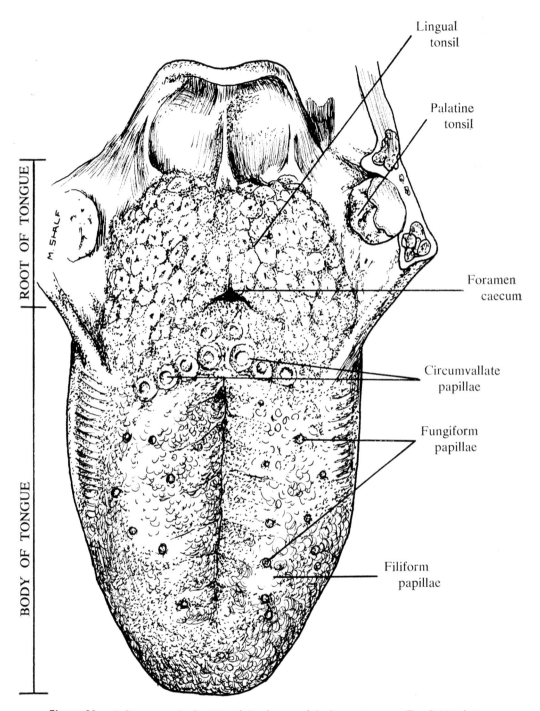

Figure 82. A diagrammatic drawing of the dorsum of the human tongue. The division between the body and root is indicated, as are the locations of the kinds of papillae, the foramen caecum, and the lingual tonsil.

Figure 83. A photomicrograph of a vertical section through the upper surface of a human tongue. These are filiform papillae. In this section the surface of the epithelium does not appear to be heavily keratinized.

Figure 84. A photomicrograph of a vertical section through the upper surface of a human tongue. This is a fungiform papilla. Examine someone's tongue and locate some papillae of this type.

Filiform papillae (thread-like) (Figs. 82 and 83) cover the top surface of the tongue and give it a velvety appearance. The epithelium covering the tips of the filiform papillae is heavily keratinized. In the human tongue the keratinization is not sufficient to impart the sandpaper-like quality you feel in the keratinized papillae on a kitten's tongue if the kitten licks your hand.

Fungiform papillae (mushroom-shaped) (Figs. 82 and 84) are larger and less numerous than the filiform. They are scattered among the filiform papillae. Due to their thinner epithelium they appear redder in color than the filiform papillae. They may be clearly seen by careful examination of the tongue.

Foliate papillae are located along the lateral borders of the posterior part of the tongue. In the human tongue these papillae are not well developed.

Circumvallate papillae (also called *vallate papillae*) (Figs. 82 and 85) are located well back on the tongue between the body and the base of the tongue. They are relatively large, conspicuous structures, 8 to 10 in number, arranged in a V-shaped line with the point of the V directed toward the throat. Each papilla is surrounded by a trench, or trough, into the bottom of which open ducts leading from the salivary glands beneath (Von Ebner's glands). The saliva from these glands floods the trench around the papilla and serves as a solvent for food substances.

Taste buds   Von Ebner's glands

Duct

Figure 85. A photomicrograph of a vertical section through the dorsum (upper surface) of a human tongue. This is a circumvallate papilla. The papillae may be from 2 to 3 mm. in diameter. Taste buds are located along the side surface; a duct from Von Ebner's salivary glands empties into the base of the trench around the papilla. This section is cut through the length of the duct, but it is a little to one side of the duct opening, so you cannot see in this illustration exactly the point at which the duct opens into the trench.

Figure 86. A photomicrograph of a section through the side of a rabbit tongue. These are foliate papillae. They are a different shape and are better developed in a rabbit than in man. The taste buds are clearly seen in the epithelium along the sides of the papillae. (See Figure 87 for an enlargement.)

Now along the lateral surfaces of these papillae are groups of specialized epithelial cells called *taste buds.* When food substances, in solution in the saliva from Von Ebner's glands, come in contact with the taste buds, the individual experiences a sensation of taste.

Fungiform, foliate, and circumvallate papillae all contain organs of taste, but they are more conspicuous on the circumvallate papillae.

Figure 86 is a photomicrograph of a section of rabbit tongue in the area of the foliate papillae, showing taste buds along the sides of the papillae. These rabbit papillae are, of course, different in shape from human circumvallate papillae, but the taste buds are very like those of the circumvallate papillae of the human tongue, and they are more easily studied in the rabbit tongue. Figure 87 is a higher magnification of the taste buds seen in the center of the picture in Figure 86. Notice the fine detail of their construction.

THE SALIVARY GLANDS

HISTOLOGY AND FUNCTION OF SALIVARY GLANDS

Salivary glands produce a colorless, slightly sticky fluid called *saliva* which is discharged into the oral cavity through ducts that open onto the surface of the oral mucosa.

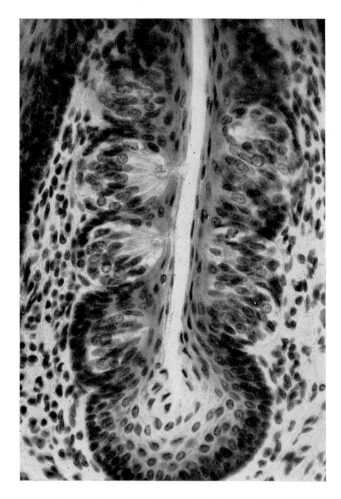

Figure 87. A photomicrograph at a higher magnification of the taste buds seen in the center of the picture in Figure 86. On the left of the vertical space between the two papillae are two taste buds cut exactly though their center. Notice the little pore-like opening to the surface.

In embryonic development the salivary glands are formed from the epithelium that lines the early oral cavity. In certain areas cells of the embryonic oral epithelium grow downward into the underlying connective tissue, and as they multiply the epithelial cells of this downgrowth become modified and very specialized and form the salivary glands. Some of the cells develop into the secretory cells of the glands, and others develop into the ducts of the glands. The secretory cells secrete the saliva. There are two types of salivary secretory cells: *serous cells* and *mucous cells* (Fig. 89). Salivary glands are made up of serous, or of mucous, or of a combination of the two kinds of secretory cells plus the ducts which connect them. The secreted product of serous cells contains an enzyme called amylase (ptyalin) which contributes to the breakdown of starches. A secreted product of the mucous cells is mucin which acts as a lubricant to the oral cavity. Besides these substances the salivary glands secrete other materials among which are proteins and salts which act as buffers and prevent the saliva from becoming suddenly acid or alkaline. Also, saliva contains some antibacterial factors which inhibit the growth of some bacteria. In addition to these products of the salivary glands, saliva which has been lying in the mouth contains various sorts of debris such as epithelial cells sloughed off the oral mucosa, degenerating white blood cells, and bacteria.

The total amount of saliva produced by the salivary glands varies greatly in different individuals, but an approximate amount is about 3 pints a day.

The functions of saliva may be enumerated as follows: (1) it assists in the mastication of food; (2) it serves as a solvent; (3) it contributes to the digestion of carbohydrates; (4) it lubricates food and oral tissues; (5) it acts as a

Figure 88. A photomicrograph of a section of human parotid gland. The secretory cells are all serous in type. In several places are seen cross sections of the ducts of this gland: they appear here as circular openings lined with cuboidal epithelial dells. These small ducts coalesce into larger ducts, which empty the gland secretions into the mouth at openings located on the inside of the cheek.

buffer; (6) it cleanses the mouth by flushing out debris; (7) it acts to inhibit the growth of some bacteria.

DISTRIBUTION OF SALIVARY GLANDS

The salivary glands may be described in two groups: (A) the *major salivary glands*, and (B) the *minor salivary glands*. The major salivary glands are (1) the *parotid*, (2) the *submandibular* (*submaxillary*), and (3) the *sublingual*. The minor salivary glands vary in size and are widely distributed beneath the oral mucous membrane.

The *major salivary glands* are, of course, paired structures. The *parotid glands* are flattened organs located under the skin of the face in front of and below each ear. They are the largest of the salivary glands, and in adult human beings their secretory cells are all serous in type (Fig. 88). The parotid gland is the gland involved in epidemic parotitis, commonly known as mumps. The main duct of each parotid gland, the *parotid duct* (*Stensen's duct*),

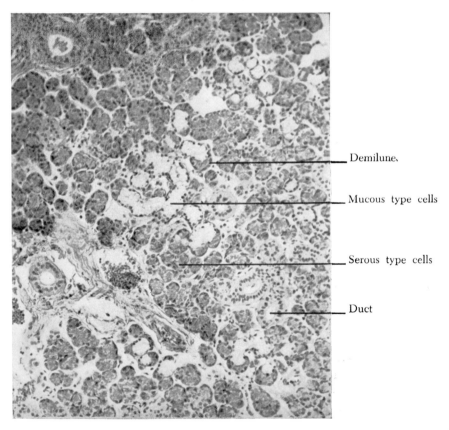

Demilune,

Mucous type cells

Serous type cells

Duct

Figure 89. A photomicrograph of a section of human submandibular gland. The secretory cells are of both serous and mucous types, the serous type being the more numerous. In the center of the picture is seen groups of light colored mucous type cells, which in some cases have serous cells capping them on one side. Because in histologic sections these capping cells have a new-moon shape, some imaginative histologists have called them *demilunes* (half-moons). Cross sections of ducts are seen in the section.

opens into the oral cavity on the wall of either cheek opposite the second maxillary molar tooth. If the tongue is passed over this area a small prominence may be felt at the point where the duct opens into the mouth.

The *submandibular glands* are located beneath the posterior part of the tongue. They lie in a depression on the inner surface of either side of the mandible just anterior to the angle of the jaw. The secretory cells which make up these glands are a combination of serous and mucous cells, the serous being the more numerous (Fig. 89). The secreted product of these glands is a mixture of serous and mucous substances. The main ducts which carry the products of the submandibular glands to the oral cavity open into the mouth beneath the tongue, one on either side of the center line. You can see the openings easily as two small prominences in this area (Fig. 81). These ducts are known as the *submandibular ducts (Wharton's ducts)*.

The *sublingual glands* are located beneath the mucosa in the floor of the mouth anterior to the submandibular glands. They are composed of a mixture of serous and mucous types of cells, but are predominantly mucous in character (Fig. 90). The main ducts which carry the products of this pair of glands are several in number, and all open beneath the tongue. Some open along the crest of the plica sublingualis, while others join the submandibular ducts and share the same openings. Examine carefully the area under the tongue in a human mouth.

The *minor salivary glands* may be described according to their location in the oral cavity. Beneath the mucous membrane of the cheeks and lips are

Figure 90. A photomicrograph of a section of human sublingual gland. Most of the secretory cells here are of the mucous type. The darker stained serous type cells are sparingly scattered in the gland, often in the form of demilunes. Cross sections of ducts are also seen here.

numerous small glands which are a mixture of mucous and serous secretory cells, the mucous cells being the more numerous. The minute duct openings of these small glands are scattered over the surface of the cheek and lip mucosa. Larger salivary glands made up entirely of mucous cells lie beneath the mucous membrane of the roof of the mouth and have minute duct openings distributed over the entire surface of the hard and soft palate. The tongue has glands in its anterior part which are mixed in character (contain both serous and mucous cells). In the posterior part of the tongue are the pure serous *Von Ebner's glands* whose ducts empty into the trenches of the circumvallate papillae (Fig. 85). There are also pure mucous glands in the root of the tongue.

CHAPTER 10

The Gingiva

LOCATION

Gingiva is the part of the oral mucosa that is firmly attached to the alveolar process and to the cervical parts of the teeth and that surrounds the cervices of the teeth.

The gingiva on the facial side of the maxillae and mandible in the premolar and molar regions is called *buccal gingiva*, and in the incisor and canine regions, *labial gingiva*. The gingiva on the inside of the mandibular arch is called *lingual gingiva*, and on the inside of the maxillary arch, *palatal gingiva*.

CLINICAL APPEARANCE

To study the clinical appearance of the gingiva, stand before a mirror or use a classmate as a subject. Pull out and down on the lower lip, and out and up on the upper lip. Below the crowns of the mandibular teeth and above the crowns of the maxillary teeth you see that the oral mucous membrane is firm and has a stippled, or finely pitted, surface. This is gingiva (Fig. 91). In people who have a fair skin the color of the gingiva is a slightly grayish pink. In dark complexioned individuals the gingiva frequently is either spotted with brown or is fairly even grayish brown all over due to a pigment which

Figure 91. The subject of this photograph was a young woman aged twenty-two years. The gingiva is firm and stippled in appearance; the interdental papillae fill the interproximal spaces; the gingival margin is still on the enamel on all teeth, making the clinical crowns slightly smaller than the anatomic crowns.

occurs in some of the cells of the epithelium. Four or five millimeters below its cervical margin the gingiva ends in a scalloped line and the oral mucosa below this line is red, shiny, and loosely attached to the underlying tissue. Examine also the gingiva around the buccal side of the mandibular and maxillary posterior teeth. The color and surface texture here are the same as in the anterior region, and a scalloped line marks the apical border.

Now examine the lingual side of the mandibular arch. The gingiva is firmly attached to the underlying hard tissue, while the oral mucosa beneath the tongue is loose, shiny, and redder in color than the gingiva. Examine the palatal side of the maxillary arch. In the maxilla the palatal gingiva blends without a distinct line into the oral mucosa of the hard palate (Fig. 80).

Look again at the facial and lingual (and palatal) surfaces of the mandibular and maxillary arches. The position and shape of the gingival margin depend largely on the age of the individual. In a young person the gingiva covers the cervical part of the enamel of the tooth, so that the *clinical crown* (the part of the tooth exposed in the oral cavity) is smaller than the *anatomic crown* (the part of the tooth that has an enamel surface); and between the teeth the triangular wedge of gingiva, the *interdental papilla*, fills the interproximal space (Fig. 91).

Between the teeth, where the interdental papilla meets or nearly meets the point of tooth contact, there is an indentation, or depression, on the crest of the interdental papilla. This depression is called a *col*.* (The word *col* usually refers to a pass between adjacent peaks of a mountain chain. In this case, the facial and lingual or palatal points of the interdental papilla represent the adjacent mountain peaks, and the depression between them is the col.) Obviously, this hidden col can be a sheltered reservoir for entrapped food, and a little-disturbed site for microbial growth. The presence here of a well-nourished microbial population can result in damage to the epithelial surface of the col and a consequent inflammation of the underlying connective tissue. This inflammatory process, if allowed to continue, can lead to resorption of the crest of the interdental portion of the alveolar process or to other types of periodontal pathosis. Sufficiently extended, such pathosis becomes a serious dental problem.

Now consider a person thirty or thirty-five years of age. The interdental papillae may not extend to the contact areas, and most or all of the tooth enamel probably is uncovered: the clinical crown and the anatomic crown are often about the same.

Now examine a person fifty or sixty years old and compare what you see here with what you saw in the very young person and in the younger adult. In the middle aged or older person you will probably find that not only do the interdental papillae fail to fill the spaces that exist between the teeth cervical to the contact areas (the interproximal spaces), but on some or all surfaces of the teeth cementum can be seen around the cervix (Fig. 92). The gingival margin in this older person is located so far rootward that some of the root cementum is exposed in the oral cavity, and the clinical crown of the tooth is larger than the anatomic crown.

This age change in the position of the gingiva on the tooth is a condition

* Pronounced *kŏl*.

Exposed
cervical
cementum

Cervical
abrasion

Figure 92. Clinical photograph of maxillary and mandibular anterior teeth with associated gingiva. The subject was sixty years old. Notice the stippled gingiva; the position of the interdental papillae; the exposed but undamaged cementum on the left maxillary lateral incisor and on the right maxillary central incisor. Notice the exposed and deeply cut cementum on the mandibular anterior teeth. This is cervical abrasion.

that is to be expected, just as it is expected that with age hair will become gray and skin will become wrinkled. Of course, diseases of the tissues around the teeth may produce pathologic changes with gingival recession at any age. What we are discussing here are usual and expected age changes.

HISTOLOGIC STRUCTURE

Like all other mucous membranes the gingiva is composed of connective tissue and epithelial tissue. The connective tissue is of the fibrous type, while the epithelial tissue, which is of course on the surface, is stratified squamous in character and is usually keratinized (Fig. 77). This keratinization causes the color of the gingiva to be grayish pink rather than red if it is not pigmented, or grayish brown rather than reddish brown if pigmentation is present; and the finger-shaped projections of the connective tissue into the epithelium (Fig. 77) probably produce the pitted condition of the surface of the epithelium in some places. The gingiva does not have a submucosa, but rests directly on the underlying hard tissue; and ordinarily the gingiva contains no salivary glands.

THE GINGIVAL SULCUS

Around all teeth beneath the coronal border of the gingiva there is a space, or crevice, called the *gingival sulcus* (Fig. 93). A small dental instrument can be inserted into this space as far as the *base* (bottom) *of the gingival sulcus*. This border of the gingiva which is not attached to the tooth surface is called the

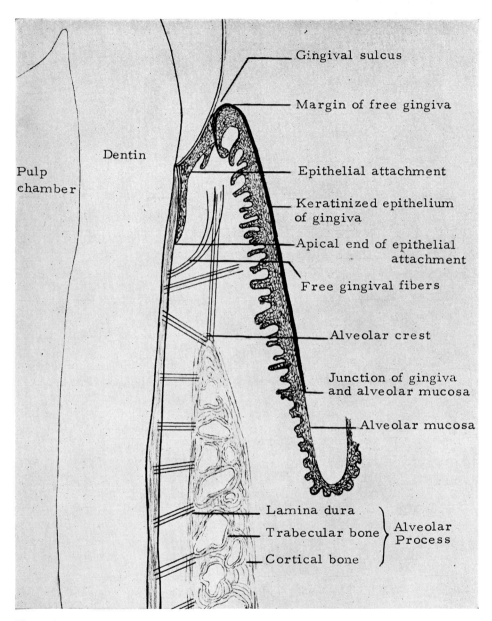

Gingival sulcus

Margin of free gingiva

Dentin

Pulp
chamber

Epithelial attachment

Keratinized epithelium
of gingiva

Apical end of epithelial
attachment

Free gingival fibers

Alveolar crest

Junction of gingiva
and alveolar mucosa

Alveolar mucosa

Lamina dura
Trabecular bone   } Alveolar
Process
Cortical bone

Figure 93. Diagrammatic drawing of a section of the buccal cervical area of a mandibular molar tooth cut buccolingually.

free gingiva. The inner wall of the sulcus is, of course, the tooth surface; and the outer wall is the stratified squamous *epithelium of the gingival sulcus,* which is continuous coronally over the *gingival margin* with the stratified squamous epithelium of the outer surface of the gingiva, and is continuous apically with the *epithelial attachment.* Examine Figure 93 carefully.

THE EPITHELIAL ATTACHMENT

The *epithelial attachment* is the band of stratified squamous epithelium that is attached to the tooth surface around the cervical part of all teeth and that is continuous coronally with the epithelium of the gingival sulcus and on over the gingival margin with the epithelium on the outer surface of the gingiva (Fig. 93).

In very young individuals the epithelial attachment ends apically at the cementoenamel junction (Fig. 94*C* and *D*). (The reason for this will be understood when you study tooth development, Chapter 11.) At this early stage of tooth eruption the clinical crown is short because the cervical part of the enamel is covered with gingiva. As tooth eruption continues the gingiva recedes cervically, exposing more of the anatomic crown; and at the same time the apical end of the epithelial attachment slowly migrates (grows by cell division) onto the cementum in the cervical part of the root. It becomes firmly attached to the cementum (Fig. 94*E, F,* and *G*).

With age the gingiva continues slowly to move rootward from the crown of the tooth, and the epithelial attachment continues slowly to grow apically on the cementum. This process is partly a consequence of the slow occlusal tooth movement which seems to occur throughout the life of the tooth. Chiefly, however, this apical growth of the epithelium seems to take place independent of occlusal tooth movement and is referred to as the *rootward migration of the epithelial attachment.* This is a natural aging process and as such is not accompanied by inflammation. As aging continues the gingiva recedes to the point where the tooth crown is completely uncovered and exposed to the oral cavity (Fig. 94*F*). After this, continued gingival recession exposes cervical cementum and places the epithelial attachment considerably apical to the cementoenamel junction (Figs. 92 and 94*G, H,* and *I*). When the cementum is exposed, the bottom of the gingival sulcus is of course somewhere on the tooth root, but it is not necessarily at the same level on all of the teeth in a mouth nor even on all sides of the same tooth. In a healthy mouth the gingival sulcus under these conditions is ordinarily shallow.

Exposure of cementum in older individuals is to be regarded as the usual and expected condition. Such cementum exposure is not infrequently seen to a slight degree on the maxillary canines, and sometimes on other teeth, of persons less than thirty years old. After the age of thirty cementum exposure increases in frequency and extent. By forty years of age many individuals have cementum exposed on some areas of most of their teeth. By the age of sixty the amount of cementum exposure in some areas may often amount to 3 or 4 mm. (Fig. 92). It is unusual to find an individual of middle age with no cementum exposed on any teeth.

The epithelial attachment has been subject to much study and much

Figure 94. *O.E.*—oral epithelium; *C.T.*—connective tissue; *R.E.E.*—reduced enamel epithelium; *H.S.*—Hertwig's sheath; *E.A.*—epithelial attachment; *R.M.*—rests of Malassez; *C*—cementum; *Ab.*—abrasion.

Diagrammatic illustration of the process of root formation, tooth eruption, the rootward migration of the epithelial attachment, cementum exposure, and cervical abrasion. (*A*) The reduced enamel epithelium covers the tooth crown and is separated from the oral epithelium by connective tissue. The root has not yet started to form. (*B*) Root formation has begun. The crown has moved incisally. The reduced enamel epithelium and the oral epithelium are in contact. (*C*) The root is longer. The incisal edge of the crown is exposed in the oral cavity. The reduced enamel epithelium (which is the remains of the enamel organ) is now continuous with the oral epithelium and is called the epithelial attachment. (*D*) The length of the root dentin is complete, and the crown has moved farther into the oral cavity. The epithelial attachment is still entirely on the enamel. The apical foramen is narrower. (*E, F, G*) The epithelial attachment grows onto the cementum at its apical border and separates from the tooth surface at its cervical border. Cementum becomes exposed. (*H, I*) Increased cementum exposure and improper use of an abrasive dentifrice have resulted in abrasion of cementum and dentin in the cervical area.

125

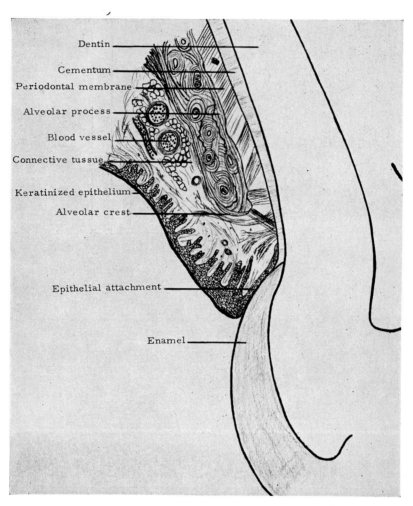

Figure 95. Diagrammatic drawing of a longitudinal section cut faciolingually through a maxillary posterior tooth and the associated periodontal ligament, alveolar process, and gingiva. This is the lingual side of the tooth at the cervix. This area is free of inflammation There is no bone resorption. The periodontal ligament (periodontal membrane) fibers are well oriented.

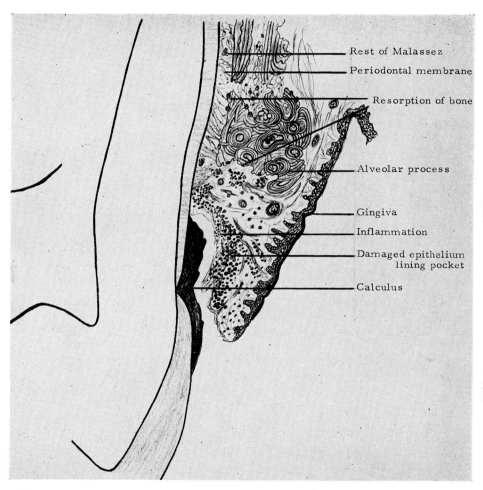

Figure 96. A diagrammatic drawing of the facial side of the tooth illustrated in Figure 95. A large mass of calculus at the tooth cervix is responsible for the pathologic condition in this area. Here there is inflammation, destruction of the epithelial attachment, damaged periodontal ligament (periodontal membrane), and resorption of the alveolar crest and of the lamina dura.

controversy. A puzzling question has been whether or not the epithelial attachment on a young tooth is actually attached to the enamel it covers, or whether it merely fits so snugly against the enamel that it seems to be attached. Just where on a young tooth is the *bottom of the gingival sulcus?* To what depth a small instrument can be inserted between the enamel and the gingiva without tearing loose gingival tissue that is actually attached to the enamel surface is a matter about which there has been a surprising difference of opinion. If the gingival tissue is not attached to the enamel, the bottom of the gingival sulcus is always as deep as the line of the cementoenamel junction, even on a newly emerged tooth. If, on the other hand, the gingiva which covers the cervical part of the crown of a young tooth *is* attached to the enamel which underlies it, the gingival sulcus may be very shallow.

It is scarcely worth the query whether the term *epithelial attachment* should be applied only to the epithelium which has grown down onto the cementum, to which we know it becomes attached, or whether it should be applied to the epithelium covering both the cementum and the enamel. The answer to this question of definition rests upon the answer to the question of whether or not the epithelium is attached to the enamel.

Many careful studies of this important structure, the *epithelial attachment*, have resulted in contradictory findings. Recently, however, evidence has been accumulating that indicates that there is an attachment between the enamel of the tooth and the epithelium which covers it. This attachment apparently is a mucopolysaccharide which serves as a sort of adhesive between the stratified squamous epithelium of the epithelial attachment and the underlying tooth enamel. Therefore, in a young person, where the cervical part of the crown is still covered with gingival tissue, the gingival sulcus may be expected generally to be shallow, and not to extend to the cementoenamel junction. Further study is needed.*

CLINICAL CONSIDERATIONS

The intactness of the epithelium of the gingival sulcus and epithelial attachment is important to good periodontal conditions. Since the gingival sulcus, despite the snug fit of the free gingiva to the tooth surface, is exposed to the saliva and bacteria of the oral cavity any damage to the epithelium of the gingival sulcus can result in damage to the underlying connective tissue. Connective tissue is not a covering tissue as is epithelial tissue, and it does not resist injury and bacterial invasion the way epithelial tissue does. Therefore, if damage to the epithelium of the gingival sulcus is accompanied by damage to the underlying connective tissue, the ensuing effects on the tissues in this area may be inflammation, swelling, damage to the periodontal ligament fibers, resorption of the bone of the alveolar process, loosening of the tooth, and perhaps finally the necessity for tooth removal.

The presence of calculus around the cervix of a tooth is often an important factor in periodontal disease (Fig. 56). The calculus damages the epithelium of the gingival sulcus and of the epithelial attachment. A series of consequen-

---

* Interesting paper: Listgarten, M. A.: Electron Microscopic Study of the Gingivo-dental Junction of Man. Am. Jour. Anat. *119*:147, 1966.

tial events follows: (1) There is inflammation of the connective tissue of the gingiva. (2) There is swelling. (3) There is damage to the periodontal ligament fibers, particularly the gingival, the transeptal, and the alveolar crest fibers. (4) There is resorption of the bone of the alveolar crest. (5) There is an increasing amount of cementum exposed in the cervical area of the tooth.

Figure 95 is a drawing of the cervical area of the lingual side of a maxillary molar tooth. The periodontium is in good condition: there is little or no inflammation in the gingiva; the epithelial attachment fits against the tooth; the periodontal ligament fibers are well oriented; and the alveolar crest shows no signs of resorption.

Figure 96 is a drawing of the cervical area of the buccal side of the same tooth. Here the presence of a mass of calculus has resulted in the formation of a gingival pocket. There has followed injury to the epithelium of the gingival sulcus, inflammation in the connective tissue, damage to the periodontal ligament fibers, and resorption of the alveolar crest and of the lamina dura. Continued irritation by the calculus will be accompanied by continued inflammation of the gingiva and continued bone resorption. Such pathosis sufficiently extended results in the loosening of the tooth.

Another important clinical problem is created by the presence in the mouth of exposed cervical cementum. When the extent of exposure of cervical cementum exceeds 1 mm. there frequently is found a condition known as *cervical*

Figure 97. Mesial surface of a maxillary canine tooth. There is deep abrasion of the cervical cementum on the facial surface. The enamel is not affected. Sclerotic dentin and secondary dentin (Figure 46) ordinarily form beneath such an area of abrasion.

abrasion. Cervical abrasion is a wedge-shaped cut in the cervical cementum of a tooth. It is produced when the person uses an abrasive dentifrice and brushes his teeth with a cross-brushing stroke. The tooth enamel, due to its extreme hardness, is not affected by this procedure, but the cementum is abraded. Cervical abrasion is seen in its most severe form in mouths that are consistently kept clean, and on the facial sides of the teeth where most vigorous brushing has been done. A study of the process of cervical abrasion has demonstrated that the use of cross-brushing technique with a very abrasive dentifrice can result in such an amount of abrasion that a maxillary canine tooth measuring 7 mm. at the cervix may be cut half through in 7.6 years; that is, in that length of time the wedge of cervical abrasion can extend half way through the 7 mm. cervix. Such cervical abrasion is illustrated on the facial side of a mandibular incisor tooth in Figure 94*I*. Figure 92 is a clinical photograph showing cervical abrasion. Figure 97 is an extracted maxillary canine tooth showing deep cervical abrasion. Figure 46 is a picture of a ground section of a mandibular incisor tooth in which there is slight cervical abrasion on the labial side, and dead tract and sclerotic dentin beneath.

Such information concerning cervical abrasion makes clear the importance of using proper tooth-brushing techniques and a dentifrice which does not contain an excessive amount of abrasive material. This is particularly important for those individuals in whom there has been considerable gingival recession leaving exposed to the oral cavity a relatively broad area of cementum.

CHAPTER 11

Tooth Development

Before the human embryo is three weeks old the stomodeum is established. At the anterior end of the embryo the ectoderm has invaginated to meet the endoderm, thus forming the primitive mouth and the buccopharyngeal membrane (Fig. 3). This membrane is located in approximately the position the palatine tonsils will later occupy. The primitive mouth is lined with ectoderm, beneath which is mesenchyme.* The ectoderm gives rise to the oral epithelium, and the mesenchyme becomes the underlying connective tissue.

THE BEGINNING OF TOOTH DEVELOPMENT

Not all teeth start development at the same time. The earliest sign of tooth development in the human embryo is found in the anterior mandibular region when the embryo is five to six weeks old. Soon after this, evidence of tooth development appears in the anterior maxillary region, and the process progresses posteriorly in both jaws.

The development of the teeth begins with the development of the *dental lamina*. The dental lamina is a narrow band of thickened oral epithelium (ectoderm) which extends along what will become the occlusal borders of the mandible and maxillae on a line where the teeth will later appear. This dental lamina grows from the surface downward into the underlying mesenchyme. Concurrently with the development of the dental lamina, at ten places in the mandibular arch and at ten places in the maxillary arch some cells of the dental lamina multiply at a rate faster than the surrounding cells, and ten little knobs of epithelial cells are formed on the dental lamina in each jaw. These little knobs of epithelial cells grow deeper into the underlying mesenchyme (Fig. 98). Each of these knob-shaped structures is an *enamel organ*, and is the beginning of the *tooth germ* of a primary tooth.

The development of each individual tooth starts with the formation of a *tooth germ*. Now a tooth germ is derived from two embryonic tissues: the part which develops from the dental lamina is derived from ectoderm, and the remaining parts are derived from the mesenchyme which underlies this ectoderm.

A tooth germ is made up of three parts: (1) an *enamel organ*, which develops from the knob-like growth on the dental lamina (which is, of course, derived from ectoderm); (2) a *dental papilla*, which develops from the underlying mesenchyme (the early connective tissue); and (3) a *dental sac*, which

* Mesenchyme is an embryonic connective tissue derived from mesoderm.

Oral epithelium

Dental lamina

Enamel organ

Dental papilla

Tongue

Meckel's cartilage

Figure 98.   Photomicrograph of a faciolingual section of pig mandible showing the beginning of tooth development.   The oral epithelium appears to be growing into the underlying mesenchyme. The enamel organ is forming, but has not yet attained its final shape.   The dental papilla is becoming organized from the cells of the mesenchyme.

Vestibule

Dental lamina

Enamel organ

Dental papilla

Bone formation

Meckel's cartilage

Figure 99.   Photomicrograph of a labiolingual section of pig mandible showing a tooth germ in a stage of development slightly more advanced than the one in Figure 98.   The tongue is not visible in this section, but Meckel's cartilage is just lateral to the center line of the jaw.   The center line is at the left of the picture.   Notice the areas of forming bone of the mandible.   The oral vestibule is forming lateral to the developing tooth germ.

also develops from the underlying mesenchyme (Fig. 100). The tissues of the tooth germ produce the tissues of the tooth: the enamel organ produces the tooth enamel; the dental papilla produces the dentin and the pulp; and the dental sac is converted into the periodontal ligament which produces the cementum of the tooth and also the bone of the tooth socket (the lamina dura).

The *enamel organ* is the first part of the tooth germ to form. It develops from the *dental lamina* as a growth of oral epithelium into the underlying connective tissue (Fig. 98). As it enlarges, the enamel organ acquires the shape of a cap (Fig. 99). By the eighth week *in utero* this cap formation is seen in the enamel organs of the deciduous incisor tooth germs. The connective tissue which is inside the cap undergoes a change and becomes the *dental papilla*. The connective tissue which is beneath the dental papilla becomes fibrous, the fibers encircling the papilla and part of the enamel organ. These encircling fibers are the *dental sac* (Fig. 100). The enamel organ for a time remains connected, by means of the dental lamina, with the epithelium lining the stomodeum (Figs. 98, 99, 100, and 101). This connection soon disappears.

Figure 100. Diagrammatic drawing of a faciolingual section through a developing mandible and tooth germ of a fetal calf. (As seen under low power magnification.)

THE TOOTH GERM

As the tooth germ grows, the cap-shaped enamel organ changes form and becomes somewhat bell-shaped, and four layers are distinguishable (Figs. 101 and 102):

The *outer enamel epithelium* is the outside layer of the enamel organ, and is composed of low cuboidal cells.

The *stellate reticulum* is the layer immediately inside the outer enamel epithelium and is composed of a very loose network of epithelial cells.

The *stratum intermedium* is a layer of closely packed, flat epithelial cells inside the stellate reticulum.

The *inner enamel epithelium* lines the inside of the enamel organ. It is a single layer of cuboidal cells. This layer of cells is separated from the dental papilla by a basement membrane.

The growing tooth germ changes form rapidly at first, but by the time the four layers of the enamel organ are well defined the shape of the basement membrane has become fixed. When the final shape of the basement membrane is established it marks the line which will become the dentinoenamel junction of the finished tooth.

Further cell differentiation in the tooth germ occurs along either side of the basement membrane. First the cuboidal cells which make up the inner enamel epithelium elongate into columnar cells called *ameloblasts** (Figs. 100, 101, 102, and 103). Formation of the ameloblasts is followed by a change in the peripheral cells of the dental papilla which also take on a columnar form and become odontoblasts (Fig. 103). The ameloblast and odontoblast layers are separated from each other by the basement membrane (Fig. 102).

In embryonic development many things are occurring, of course, at the same time. As the early tooth germs are developing they become surrounded by islands of bone which eventually coalesce and form the mandible (or maxillae). Figure 100 is a drawing of a faciolingual section of a forming calf mandible cut through the center of a primary tooth germ. Blood vessels, nerves, and the tooth germ, having formed earlier, are becoming enclosed in the bone of the mandible which is developing around them. In Figures 7C and 101 the same bone growth is seen in a fetal pig mandible.

By the time a primary tooth germ has reached the stage of development where ameloblasts and odontoblasts are becoming differentiated, other changes are taking place. Lingual to the enamel organ of the primary tooth germ the dental lamina is giving rise to the beginning of the enamel organ of the succeeding permanent tooth germ (Figs. 100, 101, and 102). The permanent tooth germ will develop slowly as the primary tooth develops and goes into function. Also there occurs disintegration of the dental lamina connecting both enamel organs with the oral epithelium. The cells of the dental lamina break apart into small groups and either gradually disappear or remain as small groups of epithelial cells.

When ameloblasts and odontoblasts have differentiated along either side of the basement membrane in the tooth germ, formation of the hard tooth tissues begins. The earliest formation of the hard tooth tissues in the human

* Pronounced *am ĕl' ō blăst.*

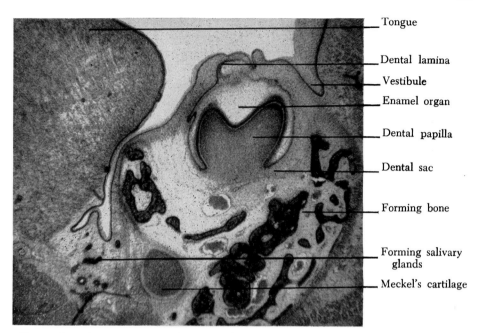

Tongue

Dental lamina

Vestibule

Enamel organ

Dental papilla

Dental sac

Forming bone

Forming salivary glands

Meckel's cartilage

Figure 101. Photomicrograph of a more advanced stage of tooth development in a section of pig mandible. The enamel organ has attained what is probably its final shape. The dental lamina connecting the enamel organ to the surface epithelium shows signs of breaking up. Mandibular bone formation is conspicuous. Beneath and to the side of the base of the tongue are small areas of epithelial cells derived from the epithelial surface just above them. These epithelial cells will become specialized and develop into cells of salivary glands. Notice the beginning formation of the enamel organ of the permanent tooth. (See Figure 102.)

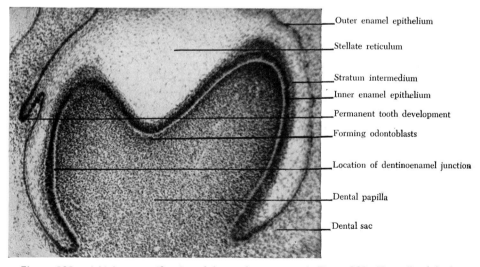

Outer enamel epithelium

Stellate reticulum

Stratum intermedium

Inner enamel epithelium

Permanent tooth development

Forming odontoblasts

Location of dentinoenamel junction

Dental papilla

Dental sac

Figure 102. A higher magnification of the tooth germ seen in Figure 101. The cells of the inner enamel epithelium are becoming elongated into ameloblasts. The peripheral cells of the dental papilla show signs of beginning differentiation into odontoblasts. The line between the inner enamel epithelium and the dental papilla is the location of the future dentinoenamel junction. At the left of (lingual to) the enamel organ is a small body that appears to be part of the enamel organ but which actually is the extension from the dental lamina which will develop into the enamel organ of the succeeding permanent tooth. See Figure 100.

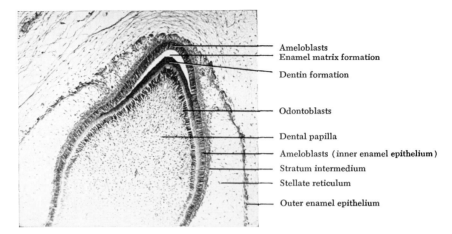

Figure 103. A photomicrograph of the tooth germ of a mandibular anterior tooth of a fetal pig. A small amount of enamel matrix is seen at the tip of the incisal edge. Beneath the enamel matrix, and extending farther cervically, is a layer of dentin. These tissues will become thicker and will be extended cervically. Notice the columnar ameloblast cells and the columnar odontoblasts. The tissue of the dental papilla here has very much the same appearance as does the pulp tissue of a young, fully formed tooth.

fetus occurs during the fifth month in the primary incisors. Dentin formation starts just a little before enamel formation begins.

Dentin Formation

Dentin is composed of (1) a *fibrillar matrix* which calcifies, and (2) *dentinal fibers* which remain uncalcified.

Dentin is formed by the dental papilla. Recent and current studies on dentin are raising questions about details of dentin formation. Until the answers to some of these questions become known, we will present the process as it has long been accepted, recognizing at the same time that here as elsewhere our understanding may be altered as it is increased.

Cytoplasmic processes of the odontoblasts form the dentinal fibers; Korff's fibers form the fibrils of the dentin matrix; and cells of the dental papilla produce the cementing substance which surrounds the fibrils of the matrix. The first dentin is formed at the incisal edge or cusp tip of a tooth, and formation progresses in a rootward direction. It may be accomplished somewhat in this manner:

The odontoblasts, which have differentiated from the fibroblasts of the dental papilla, form a single layer of columnar cells at the line of the dentino-enamel junction (Fig. 103). They start moving inward—that is, they back up toward the center of the pulp. As the cells pull back, they behave as if several spots of their cytoplasm were attached to the basement membrane, causing the cytoplasm to stretch out into several narrow extensions (Fig. 104). As the pulpward migration of the body of the odontoblasts progresses, the several cytoplasmic extensions of each cell join to make a single dentinal fiber. The part of the odontoblasts containing the nucleus comes to lie some distance pulpward of the basement membrane (soon to be the dentinoenamel junction), but the cells remain connected with their point of origin by the cytoplasmic extensions which are branched at their peripheral ends.

Now when the odontoblasts differentiated along the periphery of the dental papilla, there were formed among them heavy corkscrew-shaped fibers called *Korff's fibers*. These were produced by the aggregation of numerous fine fibrils in the dental papilla (see Chapter 5). When dentin formation begins with the odontoblasts moving inward, Korff's fibers remain in place (Fig. 105).

Figure 104. Schematic diagram of the possible manner of formation of a dentinal fiber. (a) A pulp cell called a fibroblast will differentiate into a columnar odontoblast. (b) The odontoblast has moved away from the dentinoenamel junction, but part of its cytoplasm remains stretched behind in two places. (c) The odontoblast has moved farther inward, and its cytoplasmic processes have united. (d) The odontoblast has moved still farther inward, and a long dentinal fiber has been formed.

Figure 105. Schematic diagram of odontoblasts and Korff's fibers. Very much enlarged.

With the bulky part of the odontoblast cells out of the way the thick Korff's fibers spread out, somewhat in the manner of a piece of rope becoming unwound and frayed.   In this way Korff's fibers separate into tiny fibrils which lie among the cytoplasmic extension of the odontoblasts.   These are the *fibrils* of the dentin matrix.   They are surrounded by an amorphous substance called the *ground substance of the dentin matrix,* which is produced by other pulp cells.   The cytoplasmic extensions of the odontoblasts are the *dentinal fibers*. Since the dentin matrix is formed and calcifies around the dentinal fibers, the dentin is perforated by *dentinal tubules* which are, of course, filled with the dentinal fibers (Figs. 40 and 41).

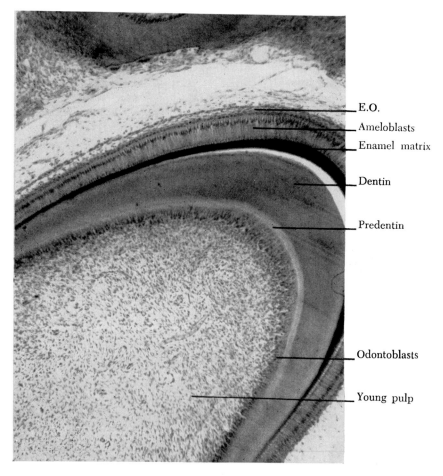

E.O.

Ameloblasts

Enamel matrix

Dentin

Predentin

Odontoblasts

Young pulp

Figure 106.   Photomicrograph of a developing mandibular tooth of a kitten.   This is a cusp tip Odontoblasts lie around the periphery of the pulp.   Outside of the odontoblasts is light-stained predentin, and then darker-stained dentin.   The space between the dentin and the black-colored enamel matrix is an artifact.   Outside of the enamel matrix are the tall, columnar ameloblasts with their nuclei located at their outer ends.   Outside of the ameloblasts the other three layers of the enamel organ (stratum intermedium, stellate reticulum, outer enamel epithelium), here marked E. O.,. have been reduced to a few layers of flat cells.   When the enamel matrix is completely formed, the ameloblasts will become similarly flattened.   The four indistinguishable layers are then collectively called the *reduced enamel epithelium* (Fig. 107).

Dentin matrix calcifies progressively as it is produced. The innermost layer of dentin matrix (next to the pulp) is the most recently formed, and in developing teeth it is not calcified until a successive layer has been formed. This newest, noncalcified dentin is called *predentin* or *dentinoid* (Fig. 106).

Dentin may be produced along the pulpal wall in a tooth of any age as long as the pulp is intact. Dentin formed in older teeth in response to attrition or caries is called *secondary dentin*. The tubules in secondary dentin are fewer and less regular in arrangement than those of the earlier dentin because, due to age changes in the pulps of older teeth, there are fewer odontoblasts, and so fewer dentinal fibers (Figs. 12, 14, 15, 44, and 45).

When dentin formation begins, the forming organ is called the *dental papilla*. After some amount of dentin has been produced the name of the dental papilla is changed and it is called the *dental pulp*.

Enamel Formation

Much remains to be learned about enamel formation; all investigators have not reached the same conclusions from their many careful and extensive studies. However, leaving details and controversies to specialists in the field, it is possible to acquire some understanding of how enamel forms.*

Tooth enamel is a product of the enamel organ. The ameloblasts produce an organic enamel matrix in which calcium salts later crystalize out of solution making enamel a hard tissue.

Enamel matrix formation starts soon after the beginning of dentin formation. Enamel matrix formation begins at the tips of the cusps (or incisal edge) and closely follows the progress of dentin formation. As the odontoblasts of the pulp move inward leaving dentinal fibers and dentin matrix in the area they once occupied, the opposing ameloblasts move outward, leaving enamel matrix in their wake (Figs. 103 and 106).

Enamel matrix is laid down in the form of enamel rods and interrod substance. The organic matrix of each rod is a product of a single ameloblast. As each ameloblast moves away from the dentinoenamel junction it deposits drops of material. These drops remain lined up behind the ameloblast in such a way that they resemble a string of flattened beads in close union (Figs. 19, 25, and 42). They are segments, or units, of the matrix of the enamel rods. This segmentation is visible as cross striations in the enamel rods of mature teeth when such teeth are ground into thin sections and examined with the high power of the microscope. The interrod substance between the enamel rods is believed to be a product of the intercellular substance which lies between the ameloblasts.

After the matrix has formed the formation of enamel is completed by the precipitation of submicroscopic crystals of inorganic substances. These crystals form among and around the fibrils which comprise the rods and interrod substance, and they have distinct orientations. Tooth enamel is the hardest of all body tissues: it is about 96 per cent mineral substance.

Some histologists believe that when the ameloblasts have completed the

---

* Interesting paper: Frank, R. M., and J. Nalbandian: Comparative Aspects of Development of Dental Hard Structures. Jour. Dent. Res. *42*, No. 1, Part 2, 422–437, 1963.

production of enamel matrix they produce a smooth coating over its surface. This coating calcifies. It covers the entire surface of the tooth crown and is called the *primary enamel cuticle*. This coating is not visible in ground sections of tooth enamel, and so it is not shown in any of the illustrations in this book.*

The destiny of the enamel organ of the tooth germ is important. As the enamel matrix is being produced and the ameloblasts are moving away from the dentinoenamel junction, the stellate reticulum of the enamel organ narrows and ultimately disappears, and the enamel organ is reduced to a layer of ameloblasts plus a few layers of squamous epithelial cells which are the remains of the rest of the enamel organ (Fig. 106). When the ameloblasts have completed the formation of the matrix of the enamel rods, they change to flattened epithelial cells and blend indistinguishably with the remaining cells of the enamel organ. Thus the enamel organ, originally composed of ameloblasts, stratum intermedium, stellate reticulum, and outer enamel epithelium, has been reduced to a few layers of flattened cells covering the newly formed tooth crown. These combined layers of cells are called the *reduced enamel epithelium* (Figs. 94B and 107).

The reduced enamel epithelium now produces a noncalcified enamel cuticle over the surface of the tooth crown. This is called the *secondary enamel cuticle*. This noncalcified cuticle may remain on the surface of the tooth after the tooth emerges into the oral cavity. There is some disagreement among histologists about the structure of the enamel cuticles.

The reduced enamel epithelium surrounds the crown of the tooth until it emerges into the oral cavity (Fig. 107). After the tooth tip emerges, the part of the reduced enamel epithelium which remains surrounding the crown is henceforth referred to as the *epithelium of the gingival sulcus* and of the *epithelial attachment* (Figs. 93, 94B–C, and 95). This epithelium in a newly erupted tooth is what remains of the original enamel organ of the tooth germ.

ROOT FORMATION

Formation of the dentin and of the enamel begins in the incisal or cuspal areas of the tooth and progresses cervically. Enamel formation stops at the termination of the enamel organ, which is the cervical border of the tooth crown. Dentin formation continues beyond this point, and the dentin of the root is formed (Fig. 94A–E). As the root dentin starts to form, the already formed tooth crown moves occlusally, although the tooth does not emerge into the oral cavity until a considerable portion of the root has been produced. If the tooth has but a single root, the dentin wall forms enclosing a single pulp canal (Fig. 94). If the tooth is to be a multi-rooted tooth, the division of the pulp cavity into two pulp canals, each surrounded by a wall of dentin, is apparent soon after the completion of the crown. Figure 108 is a photograph of a mandibular third molar from which the buccal wall is removed. The crown of this tooth is complete. Dentin has formed beyond the cervical border

---

* Interesting paper: Listgarten, M. A.: Phase-contrast and Electron Microscopic Study of the Junction between Reduced Enamel Epithelium and Enamel in Unerupted Human Teeth. Arch. Oral Biol. *11*:999, 1966.

Oral epithelium

Enamel matrix

Reduced enamel
epithelium

Dentin

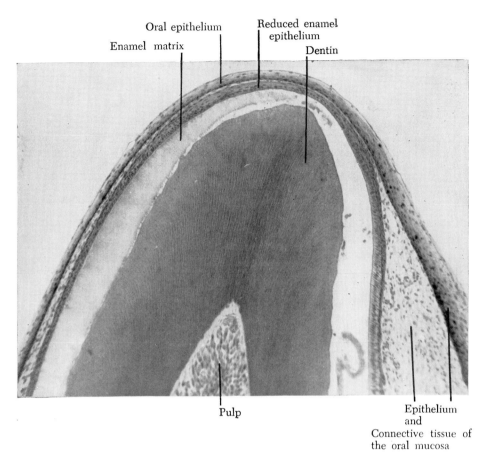

Pulp

Epithelium
and
Connective tissue of
the oral mucosa

Figure 107. Anterior tooth of a fetal pig. A little more occlusal movement, and the tooth tip will break through into the oral cavity. Around the edge of the break-through the oral epithelium and the reduced enamel epithelum will become united and protectively seal in the connective tissue. With this incident of tooth emergence the name of the *reduced enamel epithelium* will change to *epithelial attachment.* The enamel matrix on the right of the picture was washed away in section preparation. At this stage calcification of enamel is well advanced. Notice the resemblance of this tooth to the kitten tooth in Figure 106.

of the enamel, and a short root trunk is present. In the center of the lower edge of this young tooth pulp there is evidence of its division into two branches, one for the mesial root and one for the distal root. Figure 109 is a similar tooth the roots of which are slightly more advanced in development. Here the root bifurcation is obvious. Due to drying out of the specimen during preparation, the tooth pulp in each root shows some shrinkage at its lower border, making it erroneously appear, at first glance, that there may be four roots developing.

Figure 110 is a photograph of a mandibular third molar the roots of which have attained perhaps three fourths of their final length. The root canals are broad and their apical openings are large.

Figure 111 is a photograph of the buccal surface of a mandibular third molar the roots of which are perhaps about two thirds their final length.

Figure 108. Mandibular left third molar. Buccal side removed. The crown of this tooth is completed; the root has started to form. The lower border of the pulp chamber shows the beginning of a division into two root canals.

Figure 109. Mandibular right third molar. Buccal side removed. The crown is completed. There is clearly the beginning of development of two roots.

Figure 110. Mandibular left third molar. Buccal side removed. The roots have attained about three fourths of their length. The root canals are broad, and the openings at the ends of the incompletely formed roots are large.

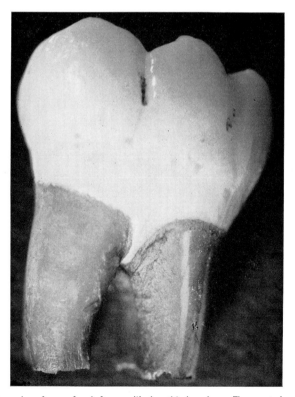

Figure 111. Buccal surface of a left mandibular third molar. The roots have attained about two thirds of their length. The openings at the ends of the incompletely formed roots are large. In this tooth the enamel extends between the roots and meets the enamel on the lingual surface of the tooth.

The apical openings are very large. In the process of studying extracted teeth students often mistake the short, square shape of such roots as an indication of partial root resorption. A permanent tooth with the apical third of its roots resorbed would have small root canals (because it probably would be an older tooth), and the root ends probably would not have this square shape.

Figure 112 is a tooth similar to the one shown in Figure 111. This picture was taken looking up into the open ends of the root canals. Notice the large size of the root canals and the thinness of the dentin wall.

Root length is not complete until one to four years after the tooth emerges into the oral cavity. A newly emerged tooth has a short root and a very large apical opening. As teeth become older and the root length is completed, additional dentin continues to form on the pulpal surface of the existing dentin until the root canal becomes narrow and the apical opening becomes small. The stage of development of the root—that is, the size of the root canal and of the apical foramen—is important to the endodontist if accident or dental caries makes endodontic treatment in a child necessary.

FORMATION OF PERIODONTAL LIGAMENT AND CEMENTUM

As dentin is forming apical to the cerival line of the enamel, the circularly arranged fibers of the dental sac become the periodontal ligament around the tooth root. The periodontal ligament produces the cementum which covers the root dentin. It also produces the lamina dura of the tooth socket. As the cementum and the lamina dura are being produced about the forming root,

Figure 112. A mandibular second molar. This picture was taken looking into the large openings at the ends of the incompletely formed roots.

fibers of the periodontal ligament become entrapped in their substance. As the tooth erupts, the periodontal ligament fibers are reoriented. The attachment of the periodontal ligament fibers in the lamina dura and in the cementum holds the tooth securely in the socket (Fig. 63).

As the tooth crown moves occlusally it carries with it the reduced enamel epithelium which covers it. At the cervical border of the reduced enamel epithelium some of its cells seem to pull off in strands which remain stretched like a network in the periodontal ligament around the forming root. This network is called *Hertwig's epithelial sheath.* Later, when the tooth is fully formed and in function, a few fragments of Hertwig's epithelial sheath may still be found upon microscopic examination of the periodontal ligament. These small groups of cells are called the *rests of Malassez.* (See Chapter 7 and Figs. 63, 94, and 96).

ANOMALIES

Development of the teeth may vary in a number of ways from the usual standard. Sometimes less than the normal number of tooth germs develop and an individual has too few teeth (*hypodontia*), or perhaps no teeth (*anodontia*). Sometimes more than the usual number of tooth germs develop and the individual has too many teeth. These extra teeth are called *supernumerary teeth* (super = additional; numerary = number) (Fig. 113). Sometimes certain teeth have a peculiar shape: the maxillary lateral incisor may be peg-shaped; the maxillary central incisor may be screwdriver-shaped, having a mesiodistal dimension which is smaller in the incisal third than in the cervical portion.

Again, there may be a faulty development of the hard tooth tissues. Enamel development may be so imperfect that the enamel is lost from the surface of the tooth soon after eruption. This condition is hereditary. A more frequent condition is localized enamel hypoplasia (hypo = under; plasia = formation), which is the result of a systemic disturbance during the time the tooth crowns are forming. This is often seen in the form of a pitted line across the

Figure 113. A supernumerary tooth (history unknown). This kind of tooth is usually found in the maxilla, lingual to the other teeth.

Figure 114. Distal surface of a maxillary right third molar. On the root trunk is an enamel pearl. The tooth was ground to a thin section along the vertical line. (See Figure 115.)

Figure 115. A ground section of the tooth shown in Figure 114. The enamel pearl is in the upper right. The roots are not present here because the section was made at the root furcation. Notice that besides having a formation of enamel in this unusual location, there is a variation in the dentin formation which has resulted in a protrusion of dentin beneath the enamel pearl.

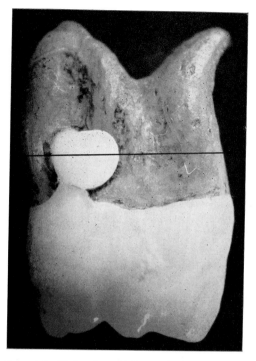

Figure 116. A maxillary right third molar with a very large enamel pearl on the distal surface of the lingual root. The tooth was ground to a thin section along the horizontal line. (See Figure 117.)

Figure 117. A ground section of the tooth shown in Figure 116. The enamel pearl is in the lower left. In this tooth there is not only a protrusion of the dentin beneath the enamel pearl, but there is also an extrusion of the pulp cavity in the location of the pearl.

facial surfaces of the permanent incisors, the tips of the canines, and the cusps of the first molars in the same mouth. It affects the areas of the teeth that were in the process of formation at the time the systemic cause of the hypoplasia occurred. If the systemic cause occurred before the child was ten months old, the maxillary laterals probably will not be affected, because of their normally later development. Still another abnormality is an interference with the calcification of the enamel matrix which produces hypocalcified areas in the enamel. This condition is seen in individuals who have lived during the first eight years of their lives in regions where the drinking water contained over 2 parts per million of fluoride. Fluoride in the drinking water causes enamel hypocalcification only when it is consumed during the period of tooth formation; and such hypocalcification is clinically visible only when the fluoride is in amounts in excess of approximately 2 ppm. The hypocalcified areas of enamel soon become stained brown when exposed to the oral cavity, so that there are unsightly brown spots on the teeth. This condition is called *mottled enamel* or *dental fluorosis*.

Another variation in enamel formation found in molars, chiefly mandibular molars, is an extension of the enamel at its cervical border between the roots of the teeth (Fig. 111). Perhaps this pattern of enamel distribution should not be called an anomaly, as it has been reported to occur in 90 per cent of the mandibular first molars in persons of Mongoloid racial stock. It is unusual in teeth of persons of Caucasoid racial stock.

An interesting anomaly which is sometimes seen in the process of examining a collection of extracted teeth is the *enamel pearl*. This is a spot of enamel, usually in the shape of half a sphere, which is found on the roots of teeth. The most frequent location of enamel pearls is said to be on the distal surface of third molars (Figs. 114 and 116), although they are sometimes found on the buccal surface of a molar at the root furcation. Their formation is ordinarily said to be the result of a small group of cells of Hertwig's epithelial root sheath adhering to the surface of the newly formed root dentin instead of becoming separated from the dentin and moving out into the periodontal ligament. These epithelial cells adhering to the root dentin differentiate into ameloblasts just as the cells of the inner enamel epithelium in the crown area differentiate into ameloblasts, and a drop of enamel (enamel pearl) is then produced on the root.

That the production of an enamel pearl is more than merely a simple matter of the cells of Hertwig's sheath adhering to the root dentin is indicated by the fact that the dentin beneath the enamel pearl in many, if not all, cases protrudes into the pearl. That is, the external dentin surface is not flat, as on the rest of the root: there is a protrusion of dentin which is covered by the enamel pearl (Figs. 115 and 117). In some teeth the configuration of the pulp canal is also altered. In the cross section (Fig. 117) of the tooth shown in Figure 116, there is an extrusion of the wall of the pulp canal beneath the enamel pearl.

Sometimes on a tooth root there is a projection larger than an enamel pearl: it has an enamel-covered crown and a short cementum-covered root (Fig. 118*A*). It is, in fact, an attached supernumerary tooth, a result of anomalous formation of the tooth germ at an early stage of its development.

Usually in such a specimen the pulp cavities of the large tooth and the supernumerary tooth are united (Fig. 118*B*). (Compare the pulp cavities of the specimens in Figures 117 and 118*B*.)

Figure 119 is a supernumerary tooth between, or in this case, among the roots of a mandibular third molar: this mandibular molar has a third root beneath the distolingual cusp. When one side of the specimen was ground away the pulp cavities of the molar and the supernumerary tooth were found to be united.

Figure 118. A. Buccal aspect of a left maxillary third molar with a supernumerary tooth growing from its distal side. When the buccal surface was ground away B the pulp cavities of the third molar and the supernumerary tooth were found to be joined.

Figure 119. Lingual aspect of a left mandibular third molar with a supernumerary tooth between its roots. The crown of the supernumerary tooth is pointed distolingually. Notice the small extra root on the lingual side of the molar.

Figure 120*A* is a right maxillary third molar with a supernumerary tooth attached to the buccal surface of the distobuccal cusp and root. When the distal side of the tooth was removed the pulp cavities were seen to be united (Fig. 120*B*).

Figure 120. *A.* Distal aspect of a right maxillary third molar that has a supernumerary tooth attached to the buccal surface of the distobuccal cusp. The distal side was ground off, and exposed were the united pulp cavities *B.*

Figure 121. Careful study of this anomaly failed to supply an answer to the question of its probable location in the mouth other than that clearly it came from the mandibular molar area. It was not possible to identify the buccal and lingual aspects with any confidence.

Figure 121 is a picture of fused mandibular molars, the pulp cavities of which formed a common chamber.

The specimen of fused mandibular molars seen in Figure 122 had only two roots externally and two root canals internally, but there were two distinct crowns, fused, each with two buccal and two lingual cusps. The pulp chambers in the crowns were united.

The shapes of these kinds of anomalies are, of course, established in the early stages of the formation of the enamel organ. Before any matrix of hard tissue is produced in a developing tooth the enamel organ takes a shape such that the cells of the inner enamel epithelium, which will, of course, become ameloblasts, have the configuration of the future dentinoenamel junction. The basement membrane located between the ameloblasts and the peripheral cells of the dental papilla is the location of the dentinoenamel junction. In the developing tooth many of these anomalies would be visible in microscopic examination of sections of tissue obtained at this early stage of tooth formation.

Figure 122. The lingual surface of fused mandibular molars.

CHAPTER 12

Tooth Eruption and the Shedding of the Primary Teeth

TOOTH ERUPTION

Tooth eruption is the combination of bodily movements of the tooth, both before and after the emergence of its crown into the oral cavity, which serves to bring it and maintain it in occlusion with the teeth of the opposing arch. Tooth eruption begins at the time the crown is completed and the root starts to form and continues throughout the life of the tooth.

Eruptive Movements

In its simplest form tooth eruption may be pictured as the occlusal movement of the tooth brought about, at least in part, by the pressure produced by the lengthening of the root and the development of additional bone beneath the root. Instead of visualizing the process of root formation as one in which the root grows deeper into the jaw, it is necessary to regard the position of the apical end of the developing root as being relatively fixed. As the developing root lengthens, its growing apical end maintains its position and the crown is pushed occlusally. Undoubtedly this concept gives an oversimplified picture of the process, for there is much yet to be learned about tooth eruption.[*]

In the development of the permanent dentition, the movements of tooth eruption vary from little more than this relatively simple process of occlusal movement in the anterior teeth, through a condition of considerable horizontal movement in the premolars, to a highly complex set of rotating and horizontal movements in the molars.

With the exception of the permanent molar teeth the enamel organ of each permanent tooth develops from the dental lamina lingual to its primary predecessor. By the time the primary tooth has emerged into the oral cavity the development of the permanent tooth is well advanced. In the anterior region the permanent teeth continue development lingual to their primary predecessors, but in the region of the premolars a change in relative position occurs. The premolars replace the primary molars. By the time the primary molars have come into occlusion, the crowns of the developing premolars occupy a position not lingual to, but between the roots of, the primary molars (Fig. 123). This change in relative positions occurs as a result of a vertical movement of the primary teeth and a horizontal movement of the developing permanent teeth.

---

[*] Interesting paper: Kovacs, J.: Contribution to the Ontogenetic Morphology of Roots of Human Teeth. Jour. Dent. Res. *46*, Supplement to No. 5, 865, 1967.

The permanent molar teeth do not have predecessors. The enamel organs of the tooth germs of the permanent molars develop from an extension of the dental lamina distal to the position of the primary molars. The first permanent molars develop in approximately the position they will hold upon emergence into the oral cavity. But the crowns of both the second and third molars form in a very different position, and must undergo complicated motions of rotation and forward movement in order to emerge into correct relation to other teeth.

At the time the second and third molars begin to develop neither the maxilla nor the mandible is large enough to accommodate them. The mandibular second and third molars develop in the ramus of the mandible with their occlusal surfaces directed mesially. The second molar usually emerges into the oral cavity in its correct position distal to the first molar. But inadequate jaw development and a failure of sufficient rotating movement in the early stages of eruption sometimes cause the crown of the mandibular third molar to press against the roots of the adjacent second molar. The result of such a positional relationship is an impacted third molar. In Figure 75 is seen a mandibular third molar crown forming in the usual position in the ramus of the mandible.

In the maxilla the second and third molars develop in the maxillary tuberosity with their occlusal surfaces directed distally and buccally. Inadequate jaw development and a failure of sufficient rotating movement in the early stages of eruption may result in the emergence of the maxillary third molar with its occlusal surface directed distally and buccally. The change in position of developing teeth in the jaws is a result of the growth of the teeth, the growth of the alveolar process, and the growth of the jaws (Fig. 75).

Incidentally, in the course of the total process of tooth eruption, the tooth emerges into the oral cavity. Figure 94 is a diagram of some events involved in this emergence. In Figure 94*A* the tooth crown is nearly complete but root formation has not yet begun. The reduced enamel epithelium covering the crown is separated from the epithelium lining the oral cavity by an area of connective tissue. In Figure 94*B* root formation is in progress and the crown has moved occlusally. With the occlusal movement of the tooth crown the reduced enamel epithelium has come in contact with the oral epithelium (Fig. 107). At the cervical border of the reduced enamel epithelium some cells seem to have broken off and remained as an open network of epithelial cells in the periodontal ligament surrounding the tooth root. This network is *Hertwig's epithelial sheath.* In Figure 94*C* the epithelial cells which previously covered the incisal edge of the tooth have disappeared and the tip of the tooth has become visible in the mouth. With the emergence of the tooth into the mouth the reduced enamel epithelium becomes known as the *epithelial attachment* (Fig. 94*D*). This change is merely one of terminology. With age the cells at the apical end of the epithelial attachment proliferate onto the cementum of the root (Fig. 94*E*). (Turn to page 124 and re-read the discussion on the epithelial attachment.)

Although the tooth comes into occlusion during the formation of the root, occlusal movement does not cease when the root is completed. Due to changes in the surrounding bone and probably also to continued cementum

formation at the root end, occlusal movement may continue, at least intermittently, throughout the life of the tooth. An important need is served by
this continued slow eruption. With years of use the occlusal and incisal areas
of the teeth are often considerably worn off. The continued occlusal movement of the teeth with advancing years helps to compensate for loss of crown
length.

THE MECHANISM OF TOOTH ERUPTION

The mechanism of tooth eruption is a controversial subject. Early occlusal
movement seems to be a result of a combination of factors: First, the tissue
beneath the growing root probably resists apical movement of the developing
root. This results in the occlusal movement of the tooth crown as the root
lengthens. Second, bone formation occurs apical to the developing tooth.
Other factors, as yet unknown, are probably also involved.

After the root is fully formed further tooth eruption is dependent on changes
in the bone surrounding the tooth and additions of cementum to the root
apex. Cementum formation continues intermittently throughout the life of
the tooth. Bone changes also continue to occur with changes in tooth function.

The mechanism which causes the complex lateral and rotating movements
of some of the teeth is a matter which needs additional investigation.

CERVICAL EXPOSURE WITHOUT OCCLUSAL MOVEMENT

In young individuals the clinical crowns of the teeth are smaller than the
anatomic crowns (Figs. 94C, D, E and 91). As a person ages usually there is
an increase in the length of the clinical crown to the extent that some cervical
cementum is exposed to the oral cavity (Fig. 92). More cementum exposure
occurs through the years than can be accounted for by actual occlusal tooth
movement. While the teeth undoubtedly do undergo occlusal movement,
part of their increased exposure throughout life is due to a progressive loss of
soft tissue attachment. This occurs when the apical end of the epithelial
attachment, which originally was located at the cementoenamel junction,
proliferates (grows) onto the cementum (Fig. 94E) and the coronal end of the
attachment, which is the base of the gingival sulcus, likewise moves apically.
Eventually cementum is exposed at the cervix of the tooth (Fig. 94G). The
apical migration of the epithelial attachment to a limited degree is a normal
condition. Exposed cementum is found in the mouths of nearly all individuals
who are over forty years old, and in many individuals who are younger.

This apical movement of the gingiva is called *gingival recession*.

MESIAL DRIFT

A number of tooth movements have already been mentioned: (1) the easily
recognized occlusal movement of the erupting tooth; (2) the horizontal
movement which puts the developing crowns of the permanent premolars
between the roots of the primary molars; and (3) the complicated combina-

tion of rotating and lateral movements which brings second and third molars into their functional position.

In addition to these tooth movements there is a type of tooth movement known as mesial drift. *Mesial drift* is the lateral bodily movement of the teeth on both sides of the mouth toward the midline of the arch. One condition leading to mesial drift may be understood if we picture the teeth in function. Since teeth are suspended in their sockets by the fibers of the periodontal ligament, they are not rigid in the jaws but undergo considerable movement during the process of mastication. This functional movement produces a rubbing of the contact areas. In newly emerged teeth the contact with adjacent teeth is on a very small area of spherical surface. After years of function the spherical contact areas are worn to flattened surfaces because the teeth have remained in contact. This maintenance of contact is a result of the movement of the teeth toward the midline of the arch—that is, mesial drift.

Mesial drift is possible because of the adaptability of bone tissue. Pressure on the periodontal ligament fibers results in the resorption of the lamina dura while pull on the fibers results in bone apposition (formation). As the contact areas of the crowns wear, the teeth tend to move mesially, maintaining contact. The slight pressure thus produced on the mesial side of the socket results in slow resorption of the lamina dura. The accompanying tension of the periodontal ligament fibers on the distal side of the root induces apposition of lamina dura bone in this area. As a consequence of these bone changes there is an actual shift in the position of the tooth socket (Fig. 76).

It should be understood that the process of mesial drift is a very slow one, taking place over a period of many years as the mesial and distal contact areas of the tooth crowns wear off.

SHEDDING OF THE PRIMARY TEETH

PRIMARY AND PERMANENT DENTITIONS

The human *primary dentition* is made up of 1 central incisor, 1 lateral incisor, 1 canine, and 2 molar teeth in each quadrant of the mouth. The first teeth to become visible in the oral cavity are usually the primary mandibular central incisors, which emerge when the child is about six months old. The last primary teeth to appear are the maxillary second molars, which appear about the end of the second year. Each tooth of the primary dentition is eventually lost and is replaced by a tooth of the permanent dentition.

The *permanent dentition* consists of 1 central incisor, 1 lateral incisor, 1 canine, 2 premolars, and 3 molars in each quadrant of the mouth. The first permanent tooth to appear is usually a first molar, which emerges just behind the second primary molar when the child is about six years old. The last primary tooth to remain in the mouth is usually the second primary molar. This is replaced by the permanent second premolar in about the twelfth year. The permanent molars have no predecessors. Since the first permanent molars appear in the mouth during the sixth year, when the primary dentition is sometimes still intact, it is important that these teeth be recognized as teeth of the permanent dentition and not be regarded as primary teeth soon to be lost.

In Table 2 will be found the time of emergence into the oral cavity of the teeth of the primary and permanent dentitions, as well as the time of the beginning of hard tissue formation in each of the teeth (see page 158).

THE PROCESS OF SHEDDING

The shedding of primary teeth is the result of the gradual resorption of their roots with the consequent loss of periodontal ligament attachment. The developing permanent successor, located lingual to, or beneath the root of the functioning primary tooth, creates sufficient pressure by its increase in size to produce resorption of the primary tooth root and of the bone surrounding the root (Figs. 123 and 124). As the root resorbs the tooth loosens. Eventually all periodontal ligament attachment is lost and the rootless crown of the primary tooth literally falls off of the jaw.

An interesting phenomenon frequently observed in children is the alternate loosening and tightening of a primary tooth before it is finally shed. One day the child reports a loose tooth, and several days later the tooth seems to be firmly attached. This reattachment is due to the fact that when resorption of the primary tooth root causes the tooth to become loose, not only is pressure relieved but slight tension seems to be induced on the adjacent connective tissue. This tension stimulates the connective tissue around the resorbed root end to form new cementum on the remaining root end and new bone around the root. This results in the attachment of new periodontal ligament fibers and the tooth tightens in the jaw. But further development of the permanent tooth soon causes more resorption of both bone and root. Loosening and reattachment may alternate several times, but as the permanent tooth con-

Primary canine tooth

Primary posterior teeth

Permanent posterior teeth

Permanent anterior tooth

Figure 123. A photomicrograph of a longitudinal section of the mandible of a kitten. The primary canine tooth and posterior teeth are in functional position. Beneath the root of the canine tooth and between the roots of the posterior teeth are the developing crowns of the teeth of the permanent dentition. This same kind of arrangement is seen in human teeth. A kitten mandible is used here for illustration because of the difficulty in obtaining suitable human material.

tinues to develop the pressure brought about by its growth will cause sufficient resorption of the primary tooth root to bring about the shedding of the tooth.

Occasionally the relative positions of the primary tooth and its permanent successor are such that the primary tooth root is not subjected to the pressure which would cause its resorption.   In this case the permanent tooth may emerge into the oral cavity lingual to the primary tooth which it is supposed

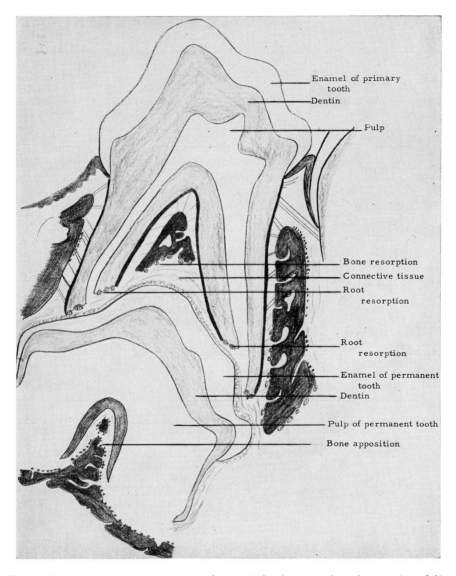

Figure 124. A diagrammatic drawing of a mesiodistal section through a portion of kitten mandible. This drawing was made from the same specimen as the one illustrated in Figure 123, but from a different section. Here there is root resorption on the primary tooth as a result of the growth of the permanent tooth crown. Notice also the resorption of the bone between the roots of the primary tooth. Between the developing roots of the permanent tooth bone growth (bone apposition) is taking place.

to replace. This condition is seen most often in the region of the mandibular incisors.

In cases where the permanent tooth bud has failed to develop, the roots of the primary tooth may resorb even though there is no pressure from a permanent successor; or the primary tooth may retain its roots and continue to function in the mouth for many years.

TABLE 2—THE CHRONOLOGY OF THE HUMAN DENTITION

Tooth			Formation of enamel matrix and of dentin begins	Time of emergence into oral cavity
Primary dentition	Maxillary	Central incisor	4 mos. in utero	7 1/2 mos.
		Lateral incisor	4 1/2 mos. in utero	9 mos.
		Canine	5 mos. in utero	18 mos.
		First molar	5 mos. in utero	14 mos.
		Second molar	6 mos. in utero	24 mos.
	Mandibular	Central incisor	4 1/2 mos. in utero	6 mos.
		Lateral incisor	4 1/2 mos. in utero	7 mos.
		Canine	5 mos. in utero	16 mos.
		First molar	5 mos. in utero	12 mos.
		Second molar	6 mos. in utero	20 mos.
Permanent dentition	Maxillary	Central incisor	3 - 4 mos.	7 - 8 yrs.
		Lateral incisor	10 - 12 mos.	8 - 9 yrs.
		Canine	4 - 5 mos.	11 - 12 yrs.
		First premolar	1 1/2 - 1 3/4 yrs.	10 - 11 yrs.
		Second premolar	2 - 2 1/4 yrs.	10 - 12 yrs.
		First molar	At birth	6 - 7 yrs.
		Second molar	2 1/2 - 3 yrs.	12 - 13 yrs.
		Third molar	7 - 9 yrs.	17 - 21 yrs.
	Mandibular	Central incisor	3 - 4 mos.	6 - 7 yrs.
		Lateral incisor	3 - 4 mos.	7 - 8 yrs.
		Canine	4 - 5 mos.	9 - 10 yrs.
		First premolar	1 3/4 - 2 yrs.	10 - 12 yrs.
		Second premolar	2 1/4 - 2 1/2 yrs.	11-12 yrs.
		First molar	At birth	6 - 7 yrs.
		Second molar	2 1/2 - 3 yrs.	11 - 13 yrs.
		Third molar	8 - 10 yrs.	17 - 21 yrs.

Adapted from Orban after Logan and Kronfeld (slightly modified by McCall and Schour)

CHAPTER 13

Temporomandibular Joint

ANATOMY

The temporomandibular joint is the articulation between the cranium and the mandible (Figs. 125 and 126). It is a bilateral articulation, the right and left joints working as a unit, and within some limit of range its great adaptability permits virtually unrestricted movement of the mandible in speech and in the mastication of food. Proper functioning of the temporomandibular joint, with its effect on the occlusal contacts of the teeth, concerns nearly all phases of dentistry.

Only with a thorough background of anatomy and a knowledge of occlusion can one begin to understand the functional movements of the mandible. It is not the purpose here to study the complex physiology and anatomy of the mandibular articulation and its associated muscles and ligaments. However, some concept of its design is necessary to appreciate the unique histologic composition of its parts.

On either side of the head the temporomandibular joint is made up of two articulating bones, the *temporal bone* and the *mandible*, with an intervening *fibrous disc* and an enveloping *fibrous capsule*.

On the mandible the articulating area is the upper anterior slope of the *mandibular condyle;* and on the temporal bone of the cranium the articulating area is the *articular eminence* and the *anterior part of the mandibular fossa* (the *articular fossa*) (Figs. 126 and 127).

The mandibular fossa is a depression on the inferior aspect of the temporal bone just posterior and medial to the posterior end of the zygomatic arch. The tip of your thumb will fit into it (Fig. 127). It is slightly broader mediolaterally than anteroposteriorly, and it is divided into anterior and posterior portions by the *petrotympanic fissure.* This fissure extends approximately from right to left near the posterior part of the fossa. The posterior part of the fossa (behind the fissure) is not involved in this joint. The anterior part of the mandibular fossa, the part anterior to the fissure, has an additional name, the *articular fossa.* The anterior border of the articular fossa is a smooth, round ridge, the *articular eminence*, which is oriented mediolaterally and which flattens out anteriorly. The *articular fossa* and the *articular eminence* are the parts of the temporal bone that make up the cranial articulation of the temporomandibular joint. (Locate these areas on Figure 127.)

The condyle of the mandible (Fig. 128) fits into the articular fossa of the temporal bone when the jaws are closed (Figs. 126 and 127), and during certain kinds of mandibular movements it slides forward on the articular eminence; but the two bone surfaces, the condyle and the eminence, are not actu-

Figure 125. The right side of a human skull. Recall your study of anatomy and locate the mandible, the condyloid process, the zygomatic arch, the external auditory meatus, and notice the relation of these parts to the rest of the skull.

Articular fossa

Zygomatic arch

Temporal bone

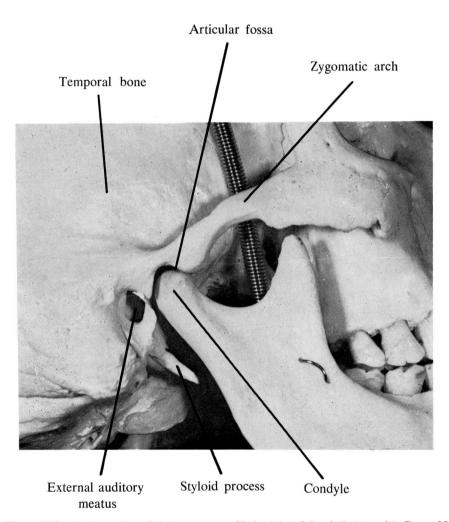

External auditory   Styloid process   Condyle
    meatus

Figure 126. A closer view of the temporomandibular joint of the skull pictured in Figure 125 If you have a human skull available for study, compare it with these illustrations.

Articular eminence

Zygomatic arch

Articular fossa

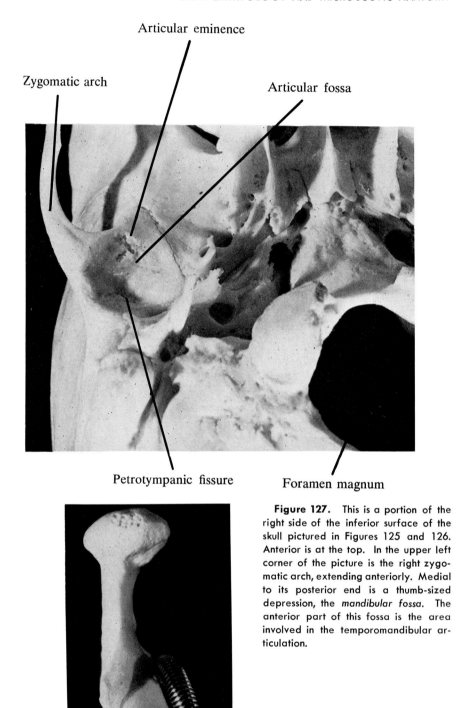

Petrotympanic fissure   Foramen magnum

Figure 127. This is a portion of the right side of the inferior surface of the skull pictured in Figures 125 and 126. Anterior is at the top. In the upper left corner of the picture is the right zygomatic arch, extending anteriorly. Medial to its posterior end is a thumb-sized depression, the *mandibular fossa*. The anterior part of this fossa is the area involved in the temporomandibular articulation.

Figure 128. The superior anterior surface of the mandibular condyle. Notice how this condylar head will fit into the anterior part of the mandibular fossa (the articular fossa).

ally in contact: intervening is the *articular disc*, which completely divides the temporomandibular joint cavity into an upper and lower compartment (Fig. 129).

Figure 129 is a much simplified diagram of the inside of this joint from the lateral aspect. It represents the position of the joint components when the jaws are closed. Compare the diagram (Fig. 129) with the picture of the skull (Fig. 126); the styloid process is a good reference point for orientation. In the dry skull there is no disc and the condyle is in contact with the temporal bone. In life, as indicated by the diagram, there is a disc, and its interposition forms an upper space (between disc and temporal bone), and a lower space (between disc and condyle). Notice that the mandibular condyle does not fit into the deepest part of the fossa, but is somewhat forward, close to the eminence (Fig. 129). The disc is thin at its center, near the superior anterior surface of the condyle, and thicker at its edges. The capsule is seen here to enclose the joint anteriorly and posteriorly. Anteriorly the disc and capsule are fused. Posteriorly the disc and capsule are connected by a pad of loose connective tissue, which permits freedom of anterior movement. The capsule covers the joint laterally and medially also, but the lateral and medial walls are, of course, not seen in this picture. The capsule encloses the joint somewhat like a stocking attached above around the margin of the articular fossa and eminence, and below around the circumference of the mandibular condyle.

The disc is attached to the lateral and medial sides of the mandibular condyle (Fig. 131); it is not attached to the temporal bone. When, in functional movement, the mandible moves forward and back, the disc, attached to the condyle, moves forward and back over the anterior surface of the articular fossa and eminence (Fig. 129). *This gliding motion is in the upper compartment of the joint between the disc and the temporal bone.* In the lower compartment of the joint a different motion occurs: there is a backward and forward swinging motion of the mandibular condyle against the under side of the disc. The attachment of the disc to the lateral and medial sides of the condyle is loose enough to permit this swinging or hinge movement of the mandible in relation to the disc. *This hinge movement is in the lower compartment of the joint between the disc and the condyle.*

You can feel some of the movements in this joint if you place your finger tips on either side of your face just in front of the tragus of the ear. First, open and close your mouth several times just a small distance and notice the slight hinge movement in the joint. Then open your mouth wide, and close, and notice the forward movement of the condyle (with the disc attached, of course). Then place the tips of your little fingers in your ears and move the mandible from side to side.

The coordinated movements of the right and left joints are complex and will not be described here. The interested student is referred to the extensive literature on this subject.

Histology

The *capsule* of the temporomandibular joint is composed of two layers. The outer layer is relatively firm fibrous tissue reinforced by the ligaments

12

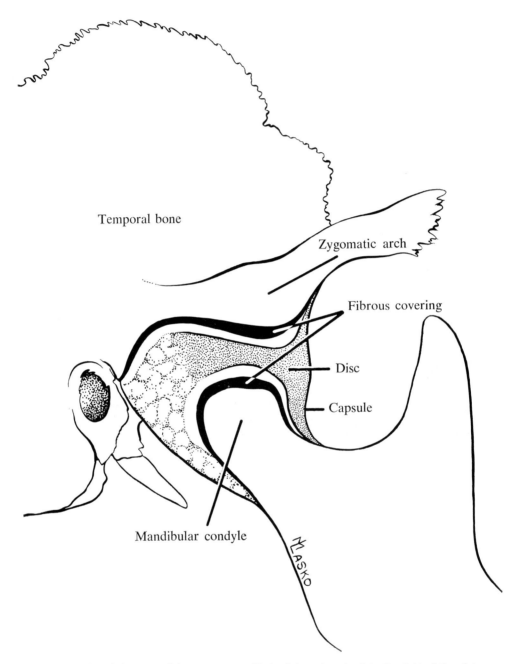

Figure 129. A diagram of the temporomandibular joint. Anterior is to the right of the picture. Compare this diagram with the photograph of the section of this joint (Figure 130).

Upper space

Disc

Articular eminence

Temporal bone

Lower space

Articular fossa

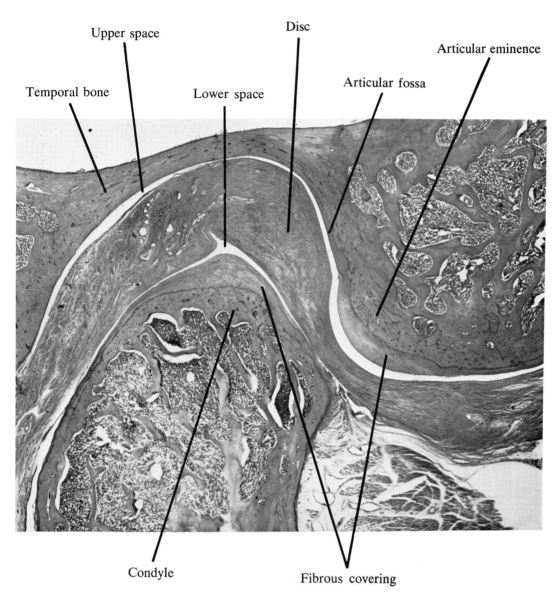

Condyle

Fibrous covering

Figure 130. A photomicrograph of a human temporomandibular joint. The specimen was removed in a block of tissue, fixed in formalin, demineralized, embedded in celloidin, sectioned at a thickness of about 25 microns, and stained with hematoxylin and eosin. This is the joint seen from the lateral aspect. Anterior is toward the right of the picture; the white area across the top is the space of the brain case above the articular fossa. The condyle has a surface of compact bone, inside of which is the marrow cavity with bone trabeculae and bone marrow. The same kind of bone structure is seen in the articular eminence (upper right). Notice the difference in thickness of the fibrous covering on different parts of the articular fossa and mandibular condyle.

associated with the joint. The temporomandibular ligament on the lateral wall is particularly effective in controlling the extent of movement of the condyle.

The inner layer of the capsule, the *synovial membrane*, is thin connective tissue and contains blood vessels and nerves. *Synovial fluid* produced by this layer both lubricates the joint and furnishes nourishment to joint parts that are without a blood supply: the fibrous covering of the articulating surfaces of the bones and the center of the disc.

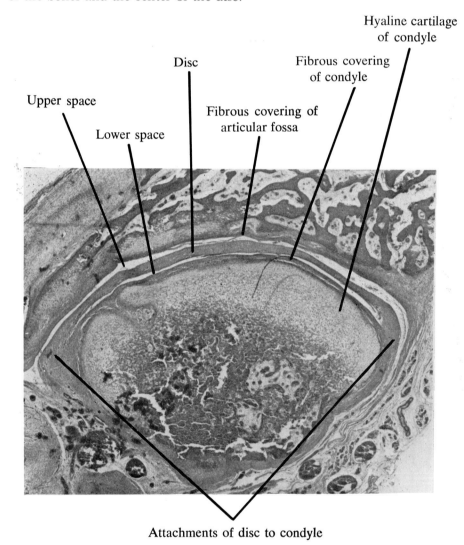

Attachments of disc to condyle

Figure 131. A photomicrograph of a frontal section of the temporomandibular joint of a human fetus about four months *in utero*. The disc is attached to the lateral and medial sides of the condyle. Due to the curvature of the bone, only the head of the condyle appears in this section. Notice the space above and below the disc, and the fibrous covering of the surfaces of both the articular fossa and the condyle. Beneath the fibrous covering of the condyle of this fetus is cartilage. This area is one of the most long-lasting growth centers of the human body. (Courtesy of Dr. Rudy Melfi, the Ohio State University.)

The *disc* is composed of fibrous connective tissue (Fig. 130), which in older persons may have a few chondrocytes (cartilage cells). Its shape is thin in the center and thick at the anterior and posterior borders. The center has no blood supply.

On the temporal bone, the part enclosed by the capsule of the temporomandibular joint—that is, the area of the articular fossa and eminence—is covered with fibrous connective tissue (Fig. 130). Notice that this fibrous layer is thicker at the posterior border of the eminence than in the articular fossa. There are no blood vessels or nerves in this covering.

On the mandibular condyle the articulating surface is covered with fibrous connective tissue similar to that covering the temporal bone area (Fig. 130). A few chondrocytes may be found in this layer, but there are no blood vessels or nerves. Notice that the fibrous layer is very thick on the uppermost part of the curvature of the condyle.

It is the fibrous connective tissue covering of the bone surfaces of the temporomandibular joint that makes this joint different from most other such articulations. Most such movable joints have a surface of hyalin cartilage rather than of fibrous connective tissue.

In the mandibular condyle of adults compact bone is beneath the fibrous covering layer, and then the usual bone marrow and bone trabeculae (Fig. 130).

Figure 131 is a photomicrograph of the temporomandibular joint of a human fetus about four months *in utero*. This section was cut in a direction at right angles to the joint pictured in Figure 130; in the fetus section you are seeing the joint from the front rather than from the side. Beneath the fibrous covering of the fetus condyle is hyalin cartilage. This is a growth center, and in this location the cartilage increases almost entirely by appositional growth (new cartilage added to existing cartilage edges) rather than by interstitial growth (cells within cartilage dividing) as in the ends of other bones.

As development continues the cartilage is gradually replaced by bone: compact bone forms under the fibrous connective tissue covering, and trabecular bone replaces the cartilage within the mandibular head: the condyle takes on the adult histologic form. But this does not happen early in life. The mandibular condyle is the main growth center of the mandible and the condylar cartilage persists, and has growth potential, until the individual is past twenty years old. It is the longest-lasting growth center of the body.

Growth of the condylar cartilage affects the height and length of the mandible and influences the shape of the entire face. The extent of growth in the mandibular condyle may to a great extent determine the occlusion of the individual: what the orthodontist refers to as Class II and Class III occlusion.

Index